YEAR
OF
YOGA

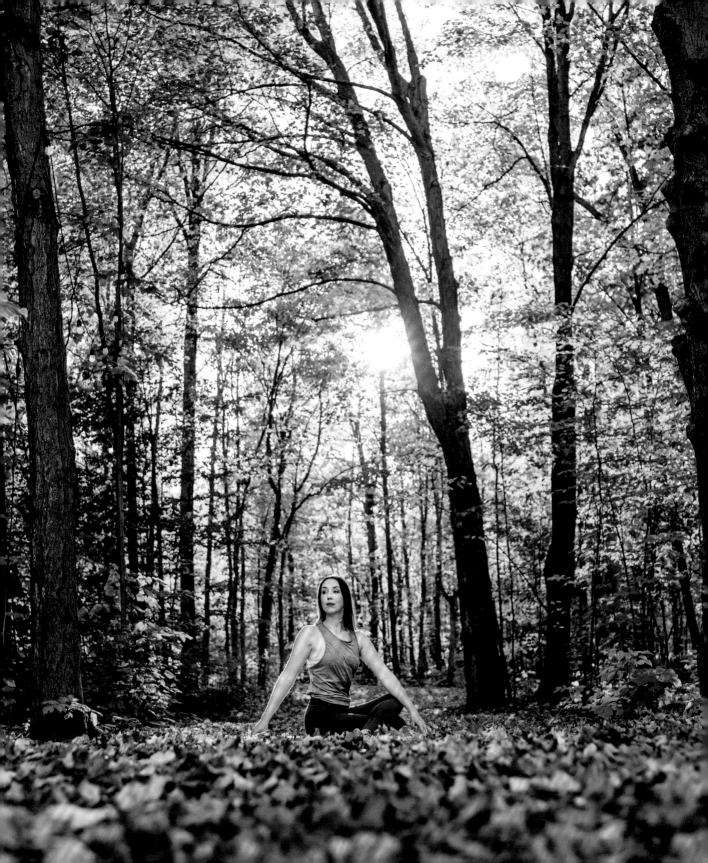

YEAR
OF
YOGA

RITUALS FOR EVERY DAY
AND EVERY SEASON

KASSANDRA REINHARDT
Of Yoga with Kassandra

MANDALA

SAN RAFAEL LOS ANGELES LONDON

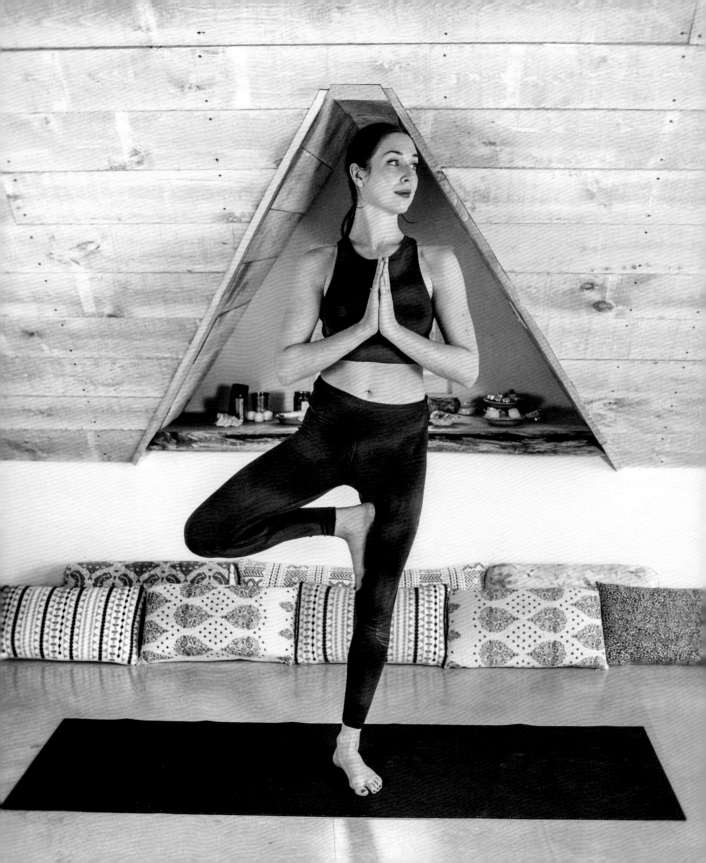

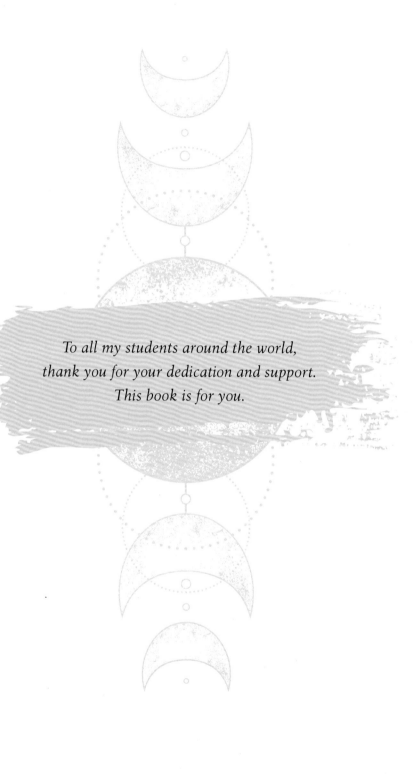

To all my students around the world,
thank you for your dedication and support.
This book is for you.

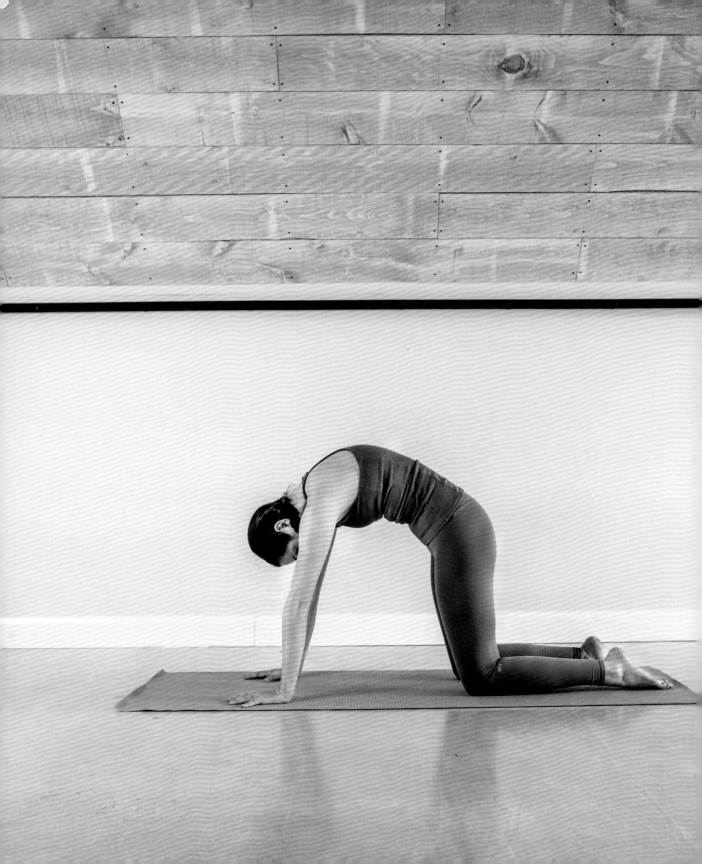

CONTENTS

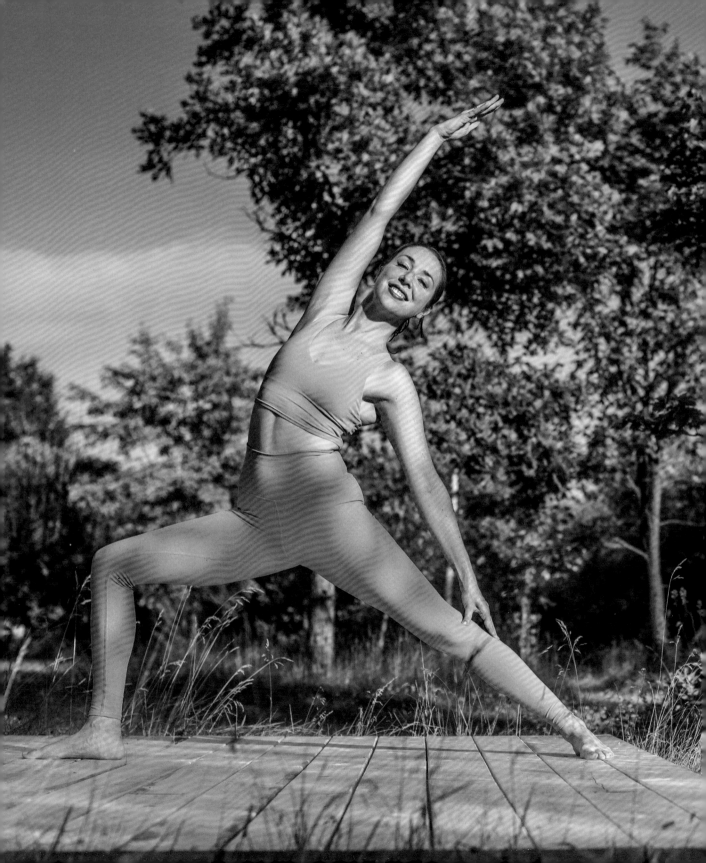

INTRODUCTION

Welcome! I'm so glad you decided to pick up this book. I've been practicing and teaching yoga for more than a decade, and I'm excited to share the tools and practices that have transformed my life over the years.

I started ballet dancing as a little girl, and while I absolutely loved it, the discipline took a toll on my mind and body. I was first introduced to yoga back in 2008, and I started attending yoga classes as a way to become more flexible and manage stress and anxiety.

While I would love to tell you that I fell in love with yoga as soon as I stepped on the mat, that simply wasn't the case. It took me a while to really appreciate the richness and depth of this practice. I had to try different styles and teachers before I found the approach that most resonated with me. The first few years were quite challenging—I had a hard time sitting still and calming my mind. My dance background made it relatively easy for me to get into the poses, but I struggled with meditating and resisting the urge to perform and prove myself. Of course, as with most things, I found the aspects of the practice I resisted were the ones I needed the most. You might find the same is true for you.

Coming from the world of dance, I was used to pushing myself to be better. This mindset negatively affected me physically and mentally. With yoga, my teachers encouraged me to go within and let go of the way I looked. The emphasis was on my own internal experience rather than on the external outcome. This took me a while to grasp and embrace, but once I did, a great weight was lifted off my shoulders. Suddenly, I didn't have to worry about looking a certain way or doing something perfectly. Yoga encouraged me to be present with my body and to appreciate it in the moment. This shift felt like a radical act of self-compassion. I learned to be much gentler and kinder with myself by embracing a "less is more" mentality.

This is what I hope for you as you go through the sequences in this book. Rather than viewing these sequences as things to check off a to-do list, try looking at them as opportunities to get to know yourself on a deeper level. The way we act and react on our yoga mat can mirror our behaviors and actions in everyday life. Notice your internal dialogue when things get challenging, when you are pushed outside of your comfort zone, and when you try something new. What is the story you are telling yourself? This is just one of the ways your yoga practice can be used for personal growth and development.

There is a common saying among yoga teachers: "The yoga pose you avoid the most, you need the most." I've certainly found this to be true. As you go through the sequences in this book, you might find yourself drawn to some movements more than others. When you don't like a certain pose, it's important to make the distinction between it not being appropriate for your body and it being uncomfortable simply because it's new. Discernment is a key element to this practice. Each pose has something to teach us, and there is wisdom to be gained every single time we step on our mats.

One of the ways I've hindered my own growth is by labeling a class or a meditation as "good" or "bad." Of course, some days I am more distracted than others, and sometimes a pose that is normally easy feels incredibly challenging. The idea isn't to ignore challenges as they arise or to pretend that our experience is different than what it is. Instead, be curious about the lesson you can learn from the experience. Every single sequence and meditation will have something to teach you if you remain open to receiving that knowledge. When we label our experience as good or bad, we can miss out on the richness of it.

We all face times of struggle and difficulties in our lives. Yoga does not exempt you from this, but it can provide you with the tools to ride those waves with more grace and

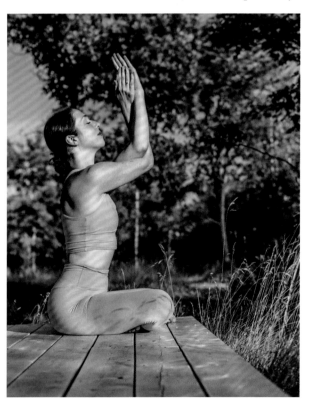

presence. Over the years, I've noticed that through dedicated practice, I've been able to stay centered and connected even during the most trying times. Yoga gives us the gift of perspective and allows us to contemplate unity within ourselves, with others, and with something greater than us.

My practice grew the most once I started to connect it with the rhythms of nature. Aligning my practices with the lunar and solar cycles allowed me to optimize my energy levels and feel a great sense of connection to myself and the world around me. Learning which types of practices to turn to depending on my mood and energy level was empowering and nourishing. Integrating yoga into my daily routine has also been a wonderful way for me to feel grounded and aligned regardless of what the day brings me. I truly believe that just a little bit of yoga every day can change your life.

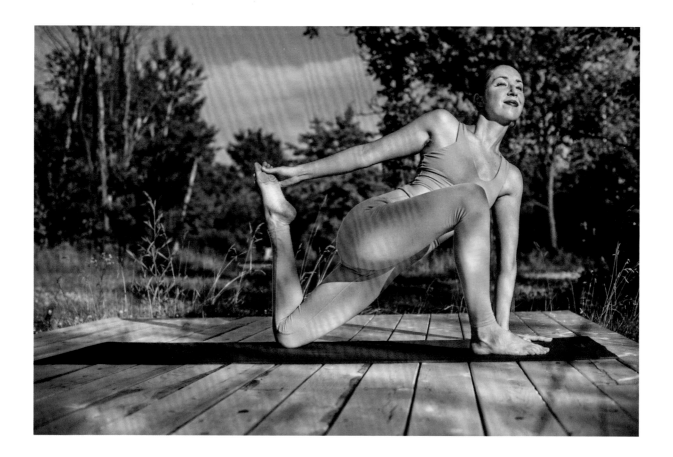

As a type A, anxious person, I've found great comfort and solace in slower forms of yoga like yin. Other styles, such as *vinyasa*, have taught me greater body awareness and helped me to understand the mind-body connection. Today, I primarily teach and practice vinyasa and yin yoga, which is what you'll find in this book. If you're new to yoga, I encourage you to keep trying if you don't feel a connection with the practice right away. Yoga is a journey of self-discovery, and the first part of that journey is finding the right fit for you. With time, you'll learn what serves you best.

My aim has always been to create accessible, easy-to-follow yoga sequences that you can do in the comfort of your own home. Whether you're practicing with this book or with my video yoga classes, I hope you feel supported along the way. I'm grateful for you and am so excited to begin this journey!

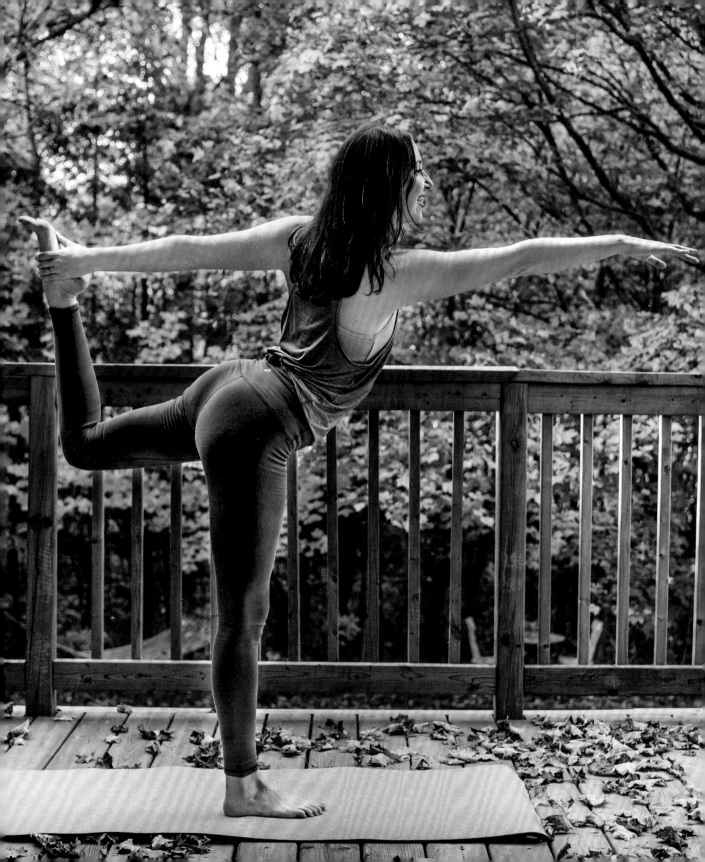

HOW TO USE THIS BOOK

The intention behind this book is to create an offering that can grow with you throughout the seasons of your life. My goal has always been to create yoga classes and sequences that are safe, meaningful, and effective. It is important to me that the practice of yoga easily integrates into your daily routine for optimal wellness and peace of mind.

This book is organized by season to align you with nature. Each seasonal section includes a morning practice, an evening meditation, a breathing exercise, twenty affirmations, lunar rituals, four seasonal yoga sequences, and a listicle of resources. I want to give you as many options as possible so that you can pick and choose the practices that resonate with you most.

You'll notice that each yoga sequence in this book has an accompanying QR code. If you use your mobile phone's camera to scan the image, you'll be able to access a video yoga class for the routine! I love teaching online, so I want to give you both the option of following along with the book and with me via video. The seasonal evening meditations also include a QR code that can be scanned the same way, which will give you access to an audio recording of each meditation to help you wind down every night.

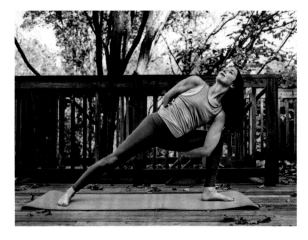

Each season has a different theme. You'll notice that the book begins with the winter season. Symbolically, winter represents the period of transition for new beginnings. If you enjoy setting New Year's resolutions, you'll appreciate starting your journey here. However, if you first open this book at another time of the year, feel free to start exactly where you are!

At the end of the day, I want you to feel empowered to use this book however you'd like. If you feel like doing a fiery summer practice in the middle of winter? Go for it! Make this your own and enjoy.

You can access all of the audio and video recordings by going to https://www.yogawithkassandra.com/year-of-yoga/

Enter the password "yearofyoga" to access the content.

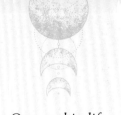

Our goal in life is not to become perfect: our goal is to become whole.

—Bernie Clark

SAFETY & PROPS

When it comes to safety, I have three key pieces of advice:

START SLOW. Be realistic about what your body is ready to do. The point of yoga is not to perform, show off, or check something off a to-do list. Make this a practice of self-care and self-discovery. When you step on your mat, do it for the joy of it. Don't worry about progressing from beginner to advanced or setting big goals. Be realistic and go with what feels right to you. You have nothing to prove.

UNDERSTAND THE DIFFERENCE BETWEEN SENSATION AND PAIN. Poses can be sensational but should never be painful. If you're used to seeking thrills and chasing intensity, this could prove to be challenging. Less is often more with yoga. Ease off of poses and resist the urge to push past your edge. While practicing, you want to feel your body working without being overly consumed by the intensity.

PAY ATTENTION TO YOUR BREATH. One of the easiest ways to know you've gone too far into a pose or have lost your focus is by paying attention to your breath. If you suddenly find it hard to breathe in a slow and steady manner, odds are you've pushed yourself a bit too far. If you're hyperventilating, that's a sign to pause and slow down. If your mind is wandering and you're moving on autopilot, come back to the steady flow of your breath as it moves in and out through your nose. Try to maintain a steady breathing rhythm throughout your practice.

You'll notice that each sequence in this book is associated with an experience level.

ALL LEVELS: suitable for everyone, regardless of experience

BEGINNER: safe for newcomers to the practice

INTERMEDIATE: great for those with some experience and moderate levels of strength and flexibility

ADVANCED: ideal for seasoned practitioners with an existing strong practice

Please understand that these are only guidelines. Each body is unique—what one person sees as beginner level, another might perceive as advanced. Your body truly knows best; listen to it at all times. Leave out what doesn't work for you.

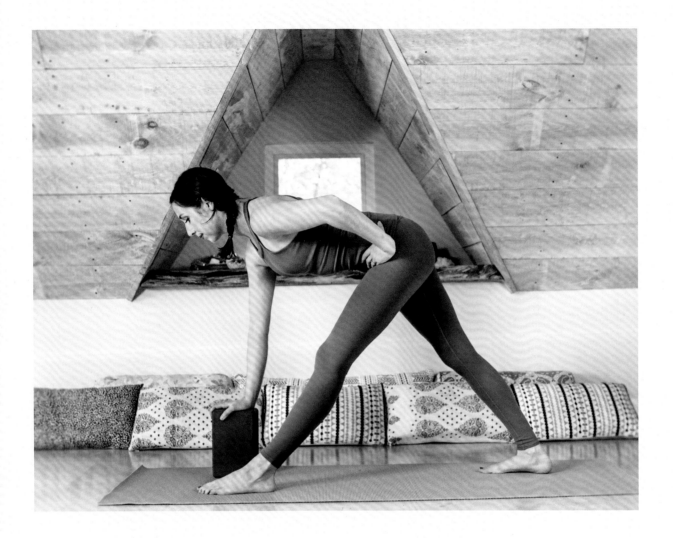

In order to make the most of your time on the mat, you may want to invest in some props. Oftentimes, common household items can be used as substitutes for props you don't have on hand.

BLOCKS (CORK, BAMBOO, OR FOAM): You can substitute these with couch cushions, thick folded blankets, or large books.

STRAP: You can substitute this with a belt or physiotherapy TheraBand.

BOLSTERS: You can substitute these with couch cushions, bed pillows, or thick folded blankets.

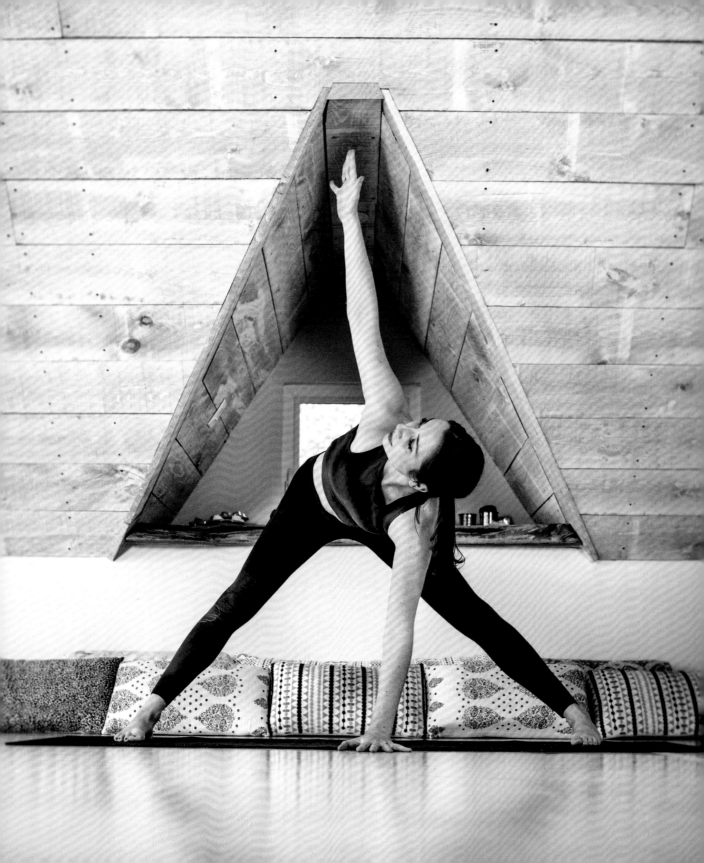

HOW TO START
A YOGA PRACTICE

If you're new to yoga, starting might seem daunting. Rest assured, it doesn't need to be over-whelming, burdensome, or confusing. In fact, it should be the opposite! I want your yoga practice to be meaningful, safe, and effective. Have fun and focus on the essentials:

START SMALL. I believe that doing just a little bit of yoga every day can change your life. To set yourself up for success, start small with short sequences and work your way up if desired. Establish a simple routine before adding to it.

FIND YOUR INCENTIVE. What draws you to yoga? Maybe it's the mind-body connection, the focus on the present moment, or the positive health benefits for your brain and body. Whatever it is, if you feel your motivation waning, come back to what drew you to yoga in the first place.

SET UP YOUR SPACE. If you can create a dedicated spot in your home that feels inviting and peaceful, you may be more inclined to step on your mat. The spot doesn't need to be big or fancy; just keep it tidy and ready to go! All you really need is enough space for a yoga mat.

TURN OFF AND TUNE IN. When it's time to practice, minimize distractions as much as possible. Put your phone on silent and ask other household members to leave you undisturbed. You can even set the mood with lighting and music. This is your time for connection. The rest can wait.

BE KIND TO YOURSELF. It would be great if we could practice every day without fail, but life happens, and things get in the way. Don't shame yourself for missing a day, a week, or even a month. Shame will prevent you from getting back into your routine. Simply get back to it when you can.

KEEP IT SIMPLE. Focus on simple movements that make you feel good rather than mastering poses that look a certain way. While challenging ourselves can be a great way to grow, this practice is about the journey, not the destination. Release expectations and embrace your personal path.

EMBRACE REST. Some practitioners swear by their daily practice and never miss a day. Personally, I like to take a day off every week to let my body fully rest. In time, you'll find the rhythm that works for you. Go with how you're feeling and don't push yourself.

Yoga is not about touching your toes. It is what you learn on the way down.

—Jigar Gor

HOW TO ENHANCE A YOGA PRACTICE

It's normal to become uninspired by a yoga practice over time. If you find yourself practicing on autopilot or stuck in a rut, here are some tips and techniques that have helped me to get reinspired.

SET AN INTENTION. Yoga can be like a moving meditation and an act of devotion. Before you begin, close your eyes and ask yourself the following questions:

- Why am I stepping on my mat today?
- What motivates me to practice?
- What does this practice have to teach me?

While intentions can be focused on the physical, see if you can peel back the layers and find deeper meaning from your time on the mat. How does it support your emotional, mental, and spiritual health? Let this be your guide and motivation, and aim to weave each pose with mindful intent and awareness.

READ ABOUT IT. Yoga is first and foremost a spiritual practice and philosophy. Much of the work happens internally through *svadhyaya*, self-study and contemplation. If you're craving deeper meaning and connection, I encourage you to read some of yoga's sacred texts as part of your daily ritual. You'll find reading recommendations throughout this book that can help you enhance and elevate your practice.

EXPLORE THE EIGHT LIMBS OF YOGA. *The Yoga Sutras of Patanjali* provides tools and guidelines to living a life in harmony with the world, ourselves, and the divine. In this text, the eight limbs of yoga are defined:

Yama: restraints
Niyama: observances
Asana: posture
Pranayama: breath control
Pratyahara: sensory withdrawal
Dharana: concentration
Dhyana: meditation
Samadhi: union or bliss

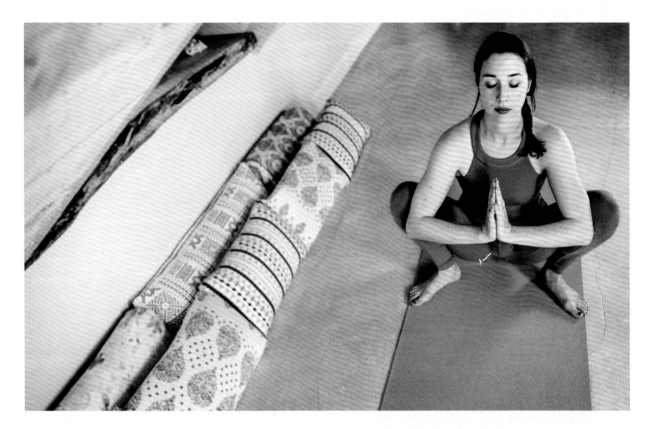

In *Year of Yoga*, we'll explore a few of these limbs, such as *asana*, *pranayama*, and *dhyana*, but the richness of yoga comes from the entirety of its system. To get the most out of your practice, spend some time studying the other limbs.

CLOSE YOUR EYES. Another great way to enhance your time on the mat is by practicing with your eyes closed. This might sound daunting, but it's an excellent way to really feel your body and connect with your breath. When your eyes are closed, you have to rely on your other senses to guide you. It also adds an extra layer of difficulty to your movements and can push you out of your comfort zone, which is an amazing way to grow and learn. Of course, always make safety a priority and only do this if it is suitable for you.

GO OUTSIDE. You might notice that many *asanas,* or yoga poses, are named after animals, landscapes, and other elements of nature. *Tadasana*, Mountain pose, *Garudasana*, Eagle pose, and *Vrksasana*, Tree pose, are just a few examples. Personally, there's nothing that inspires me more than the great outdoors. Infuse your practice with a fresh new perspective by bringing your yoga mat outside and letting nature be your guide.

VINYASA

In many of the sequences outlined in this book, you'll notice the term *vinyasa*—meaning "to place in a special way"—frequently written as an instruction. A vinyasa consists of the following four yoga poses performed in order, with one breath per pose.

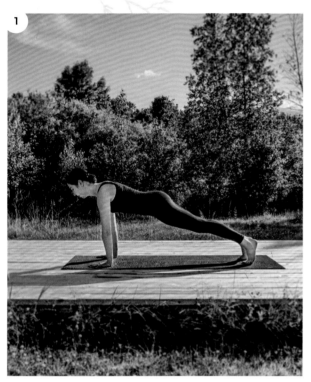

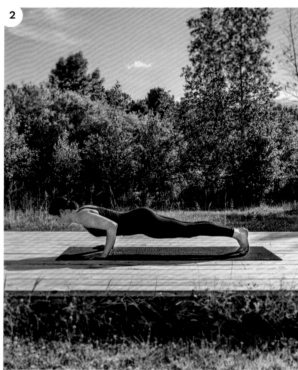

1. Plank Pose (*Kumbhakasana*)

Place yourself in a Plank position by aligning your shoulders over your wrists and straightening your legs. Push down into your fingertips and broaden through your upper back. Create a straight diagonal line with your head, hips, and heels. Engage your abdominal muscles and hug your upper arms toward one another. Hold for one inhale.

2. Four-Limbed Staff Pose

(*Chaturanga Dandasana*)

Exhale and rock forward onto the tips of your toes as you bend your elbows and lower halfway down. Hug your elbows toward your rib cage and keep them aligned over your wrists at a 90-degree angle. You can make this pose easier by lowering your knees to the mat.

Yoga is not a work-out, it is a work-in. And this is the point of spiritual practice; to make us teachable; to open up our hearts and focus our awareness so that we can know what we already know and be who we already are.

—Rolf Gates

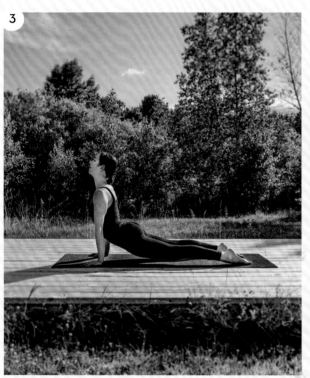

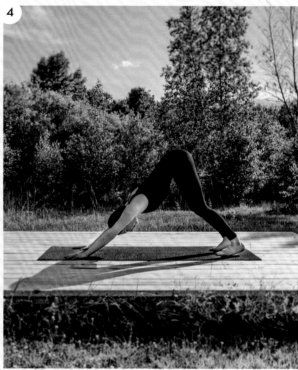

3. Upward-Facing Dog Pose

(*Urdhva Mukha Svanasana*)

Inhale and straighten your arms as you untuck your toes to come into a backbend. Push into the tops of your feet and roll your shoulders back to open your chest. Your hips should be lifted off the floor as you hug your inner thighs toward one another and lengthen your spine.

4. Downward-Facing Dog Pose

(*Adho Mukha Svanasana*)

Exhale and tuck your toes, using core strength to lift your hips up and back. Reach your chest toward your thighs and press your heels toward the mat. Bend your knees as much as needed. Draw your lower belly in to engage your abdominal muscles and curl your tailbone up toward the sky.

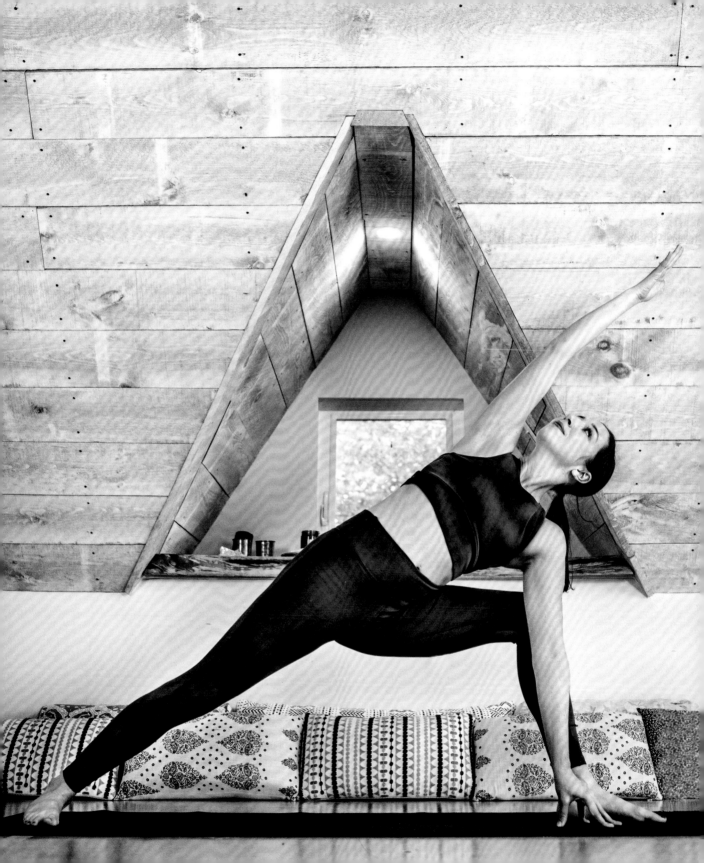

LUNAR PRACTICES

The phases of the moon allow us to reflect and attune to the phases of our lives. Connecting to this monthly cycle with yoga practices calls up the inherent wisdom of nature that is inside us. There are eight phases of the moon, but we'll focus on the two contrasting ones: the new moon and the full moon.

The new moon is the beginning of everything, for everything begins in the dark. It gives us the beautiful gift of starting fresh every month. This is the most powerful time to dream, set intentions, visualize, and practice self-care.

The full moon happens roughly fourteen days after the new moon and is the brightest moon of the month. It lights up the sky and lights up our hearts with its invitation to celebrate and recognize the abundance already present in our lives.

I recommend practicing these sequences at night with very few distractions. If the weather permits, practice outdoors accompanied by the recommended lunar playlist. Turn your phone off, grab your journal, light a few candles, and get focused.

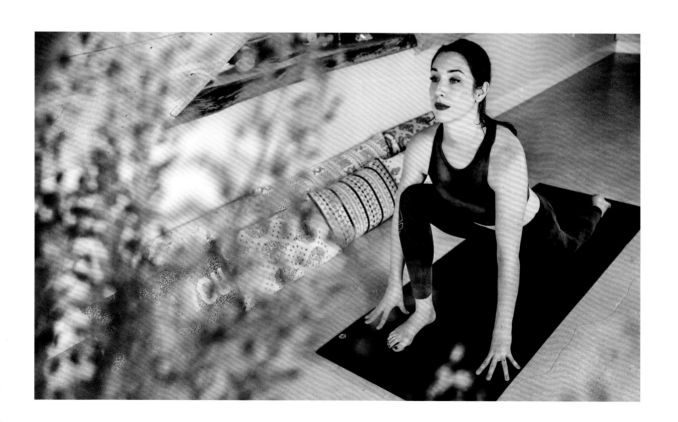

NEW MOON LISTICLE

 ## Music

"Small Memory" by Jon Hopkins

"Beacon" by Ayla Nereo

"Jai Ma" by Govind Das and Radha

"Wish You Were Here" by Pink Floyd

"Higher Love" by James Vincent McMorrow

"When I Get My Hands on You" by The New Basement Tapes

"Lullaby" by Trevor Hall

"Heavy Rope (Acoustic)" by Lights

"Mother of the Water" by Alexa Sunshine Rose

"Om Mani Padme Hum" by Veet Vichara & Premanjali

"Deep Peace" by Ashana

"Opening the Heart" by Annie Jameson

 ## Books

Moon Time by Lucy H. Pearce

Women Who Run with the Wolves by Clarissa Pinkola Estés

Moonology by Yasmin Boland

 ## Crystals

CLEAR QUARTZ: When it comes to setting intentions, clear quartz is the way to go! This stone amplifies energy and clarifies your thoughts. It is sometimes referred to as the master healer.

BLACK TOURMALINE: This crystal represents the darkness of the new moon. Use this stone to uncover hidden parts of yourself. It can be used for deep healing and grounding.

 ## Scents & Oils

SAGE: Sage has long been regarded as an energetically cleansing plant by various cultures around the world, from the ancient Romans to the Celts and Indigenous populations across North America. Use it for new beginnings and to shift your mood.

CEDARWOOD: If you're feeling frazzled or distracted, cedarwood can help ground you and calm your nerves.

FULL MOON LISTICLE

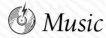 ## Music

"Please Prepare Me" by Beautiful Chorus
"Veiled Grey" by Christian Löffler
"Harvest Moon" by Neil Young
"Blessed We Are" by Peia
"Crystal" by Stevie Nicks
"Slowly" by Max Sedgley
"Pressure" by Milk & Bone
"Fly Me to the Moon" by Minnie Driver
"Goodnight Moon Child" by Beautiful Chorus
"Lakshmi Mantra" by Jaya Lakshmi and
    Ananda
"The Sound of Silence" by Pat Metheny

 ## Books

Lunar Abundance by Ezzie Spencer
Awakening Shakti by Sally Kempton
Yoga Poems by Leza Lowitz

 ## Crystals

MOONSTONE: This crystal can help you tap into your highest vision and intuition. It is also thought to bring about good dreams.

SELENITE: Named after the ancient Greek goddess of the moon, Selene, selenite is the perfect full moon ally. It is an energetic cleanser connected to higher consciousness.

 ## Scents & Oils

VANILLA: Embrace the vibrancy and sensuality of the full moon with this natural aphrodisiac. Vanilla can also be a mood booster.

YLANG YLANG: Use this scent to connect with your divine feminine energy. It also relates to serenity and joy.

NEW MOON YIN YOGA FLOW

LEVEL: All Levels   **PROPS REQUIRED:** 2 blocks

Use this deeply restorative yin yoga sequence to set your intention for the upcoming lunar cycle.

Yin yoga is a passive practice where we focus on the fascia and deep connective tissues. Try to relax your muscles as you hold the poses for three to five minutes on each side. Remember not to push or force yourself into the pose—less is more.

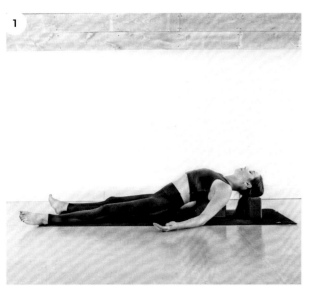

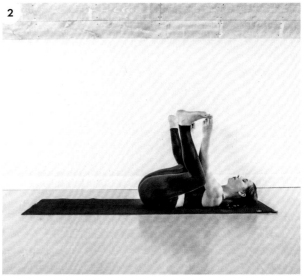

1. Supported Fish Pose

Lie back on two blocks so that they support your head and upper back, right between your shoulder blades. The blocks can be on their lowest or middle level, whichever one is most comfortable to you. Relax your arms by your sides and extend your legs out. Feel your rib cage expand with every breath you take and connect to your heart space. Hold for three to five minutes before coming out of the pose slowly and mindfully.

2. Happy Baby Pose

Move your blocks off to the side and lie back on your mat. Draw your knees in toward your shoulders and press your tailbone into the floor. Stay here or progress into the full version of the pose by stacking your ankles over your knees and holding on to your big toes. Hold for three to five minutes.

Throughout your practice, tune in to your innermost desires and notice what thoughts and emotions come up for you. As we release physical tension from our bodies, it becomes easier to release mental and emotional tension as well.

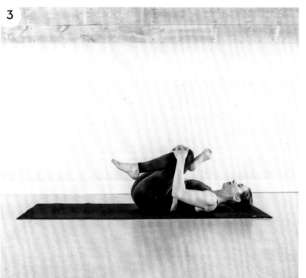

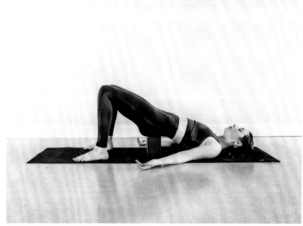

3. Reclined Swan Pose

Bring your feet flat to the floor with your knees bent. Cross your right ankle over the top of your left thigh and flex your right foot. Thread your arms through your legs to grab the back of your left thigh or the front of your left shin. Draw your left thigh in toward your chest to stretch into your right hip. Hold the pose for three to five minutes before repeating on the second side.

4. Supported Bridge Pose

Place your feet flat on the floor with your knees bent and grab one of your blocks. Lift your hips up and slide the block under your seat. Your block can be on the lowest or middle level, whichever one is most comfortable for you. Make sure your block is under your tailbone rather than your lower back. Relax your arms by your sides and choose to either keep your knees bent or extend your legs straight for a deeper stretch. Hold for three to five minutes.

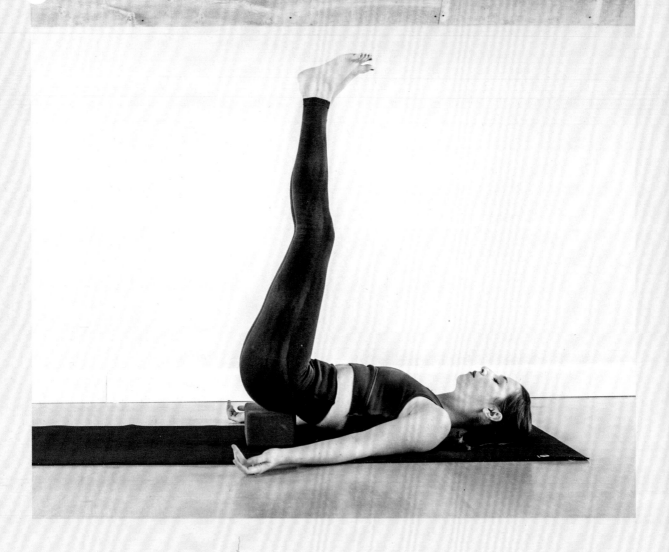

5. Waterfall Pose

If you had your legs extended, slowly walk your feet back so they are flat on the floor. Place your block on its lowest level and lift your legs up toward the sky. Keep your arms by your sides or extend them up overhead for a gentle stretch in your upper body. Stay in this inversion for three to five minutes before easing out.

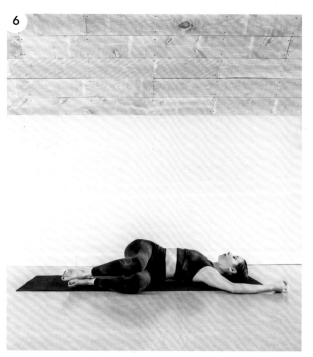

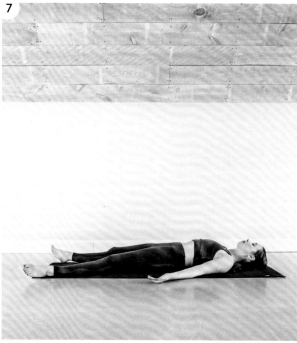

6. Lying Spinal Twist Pose

Bring your feet back to the floor and move your block out to the side. Open your arms into a cactus shape with your elbows bent at a 90-degree angle. Lift your hips up and move them a few inches to the right before lowering your knees and thighs over to the left. Keep your head neutral or turn it to look over your right shoulder for a deeper twist. Hold for three to five minutes before repeating on the second side.

7. Corpse Pose

Extend your legs out one at a time, bringing your feet toward the corners of your mat. Soften your shoulders away from your ears as you relax your arms by your sides with your palms facing up. Close your eyes and breathe deeply, holding the pose for five minutes or longer.

When you're ready to close your practice, take your time to sit up and resume your evening. You might grab a journal and write down any insights from your experience. You can also use the following prompts to guide your thoughts:

- What is my intention for this new moon?
- What is one word that describes how I want to feel?
- What is important to me right now?
- What am I needing more of in my life?

FULL MOON YOGA FLOW

LEVEL: Beginner to Intermediate   **PROPS REQUIRED:** Block (optional)

Use this full moon yoga flow to focus on abundance, gratitude, and optimism. As you move and breathe, acknowledge all the ways your new moon intention has manifested this month and celebrate the fullness of your life. This is a slow flow with a strong emphasis on opening up your hips.

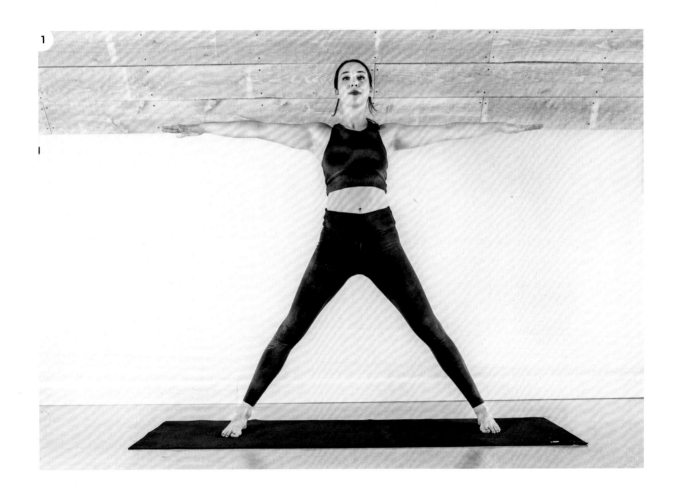

1. Five-Pointed Star Pose (*Utthita Tadasana*)
Begin standing with your legs wide apart. Align your feet parallel to the short edges of your mat. Reach your arms out parallel to the ground and lengthen your spine. Take five deep breaths here.

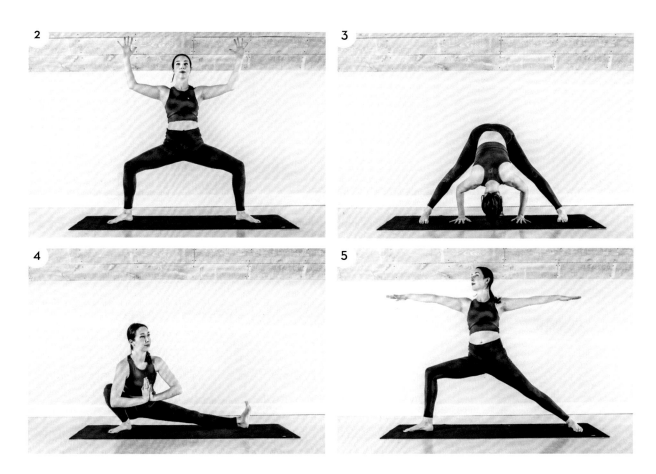

2. Goddess Pose (*Utkata Konasana*)

From Five-Pointed Star pose, turn your heels in so your feet are at a 45-degree angle. Bend your knees into a deep squat and bend your elbows at a 90-degree angle. Draw your low belly in and stay here for ten deep breaths.

4. Side Lunge Pose (*Skandasana*)

Turn your heels in so your feet are at a 45-degree angle. Bend your right knee as much as you can while keeping your left leg straight, and walk your hands over to the right. Rest your hands on a block or the mat or bring your hands to your heart in prayer. Hold for five breaths before switching sides and repeating both sides three times.

3. Wide-Legged Forward Bend Pose

(*Prasarita Padottanasana*)

Straighten your legs and realign your feet so they are parallel to the shorter edges of your mat. Bring your hands to your hips and hinge forward to fold down. Choose to place your hands on a block or the mat or reach for your big toes. Hold for ten breaths.

5. Warrior 2 Pose (*Virabhadrasana II*)

Come back through your Wide-Legged Forward Bend pose and lift your torso all the way up. Turn your right foot to point toward the top of the mat and align your left foot parallel to the back of your mat. Bend your right knee generously and extend your arms out, palms facing down. Gaze over your right hand and hold for ten breaths before switching sides.

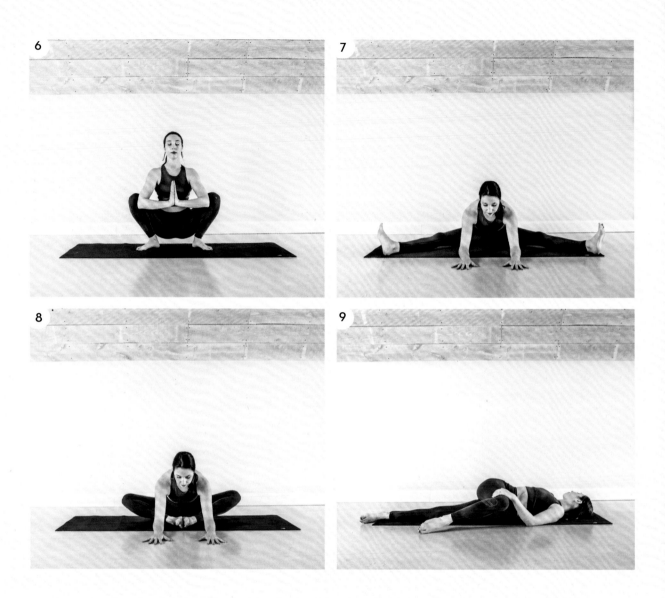

6. Garland Pose (*Malasana*)

Straighten your legs and bring your feet in so they are hip-width apart with your toes pointed out at a 45-degree angle. Sit all the way down into a squat position. You can sit on your block to make the pose easier. Bring your hands in prayer at your heart and use your elbows to press your knees wider. Lengthen your spine and hold for ten breaths.

7. Wide-Angle Seated Forward Bend Pose (*Upavistha Konasana*)

Come all the way down to sitting and open your legs as wide as is comfortable. You can sit on a block or directly on your mat. Fold forward by hinging from your hips and reach your arms out in front of you. Hold for twenty breaths.

8. Butterfly Pose (*Baddha Konasana*)

Lift your chest back up and bend your knees to bring the soles of your feet together. You can sit on a block or directly on your mat. Fold forward and extend your arms out or hold on to your big toes with your index and middle fingers. Hold for twenty breaths.

9. Reclined Spinal Twist Pose
(*Supta Matsyendrasana*)

Come out of Butterfly pose and lower all the way down to your back. Pull your right knee in to your chest and extend your left leg straight. Cross your right thigh over your chest with the help of your left hand and extend your right arm out to the side. Gaze over your right shoulder and hold for ten breaths before switching sides.

10

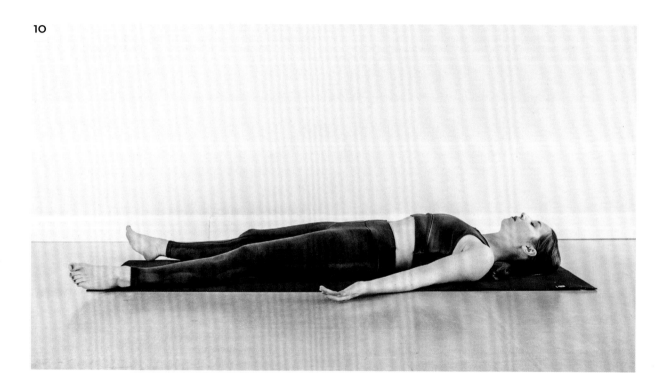

10. Corpse Pose (*Savasana*)

Release the twist and extend your arms and legs out. Soften your shoulders away from your ears, turn your palms upward, close your eyes, and breathe deeply. Stay for five minutes or longer.

After your practice, take the time to journal and answer the following prompts:

What am I most grateful for right now?
How has abundance shown up for me lately?
What lessons have I learned?

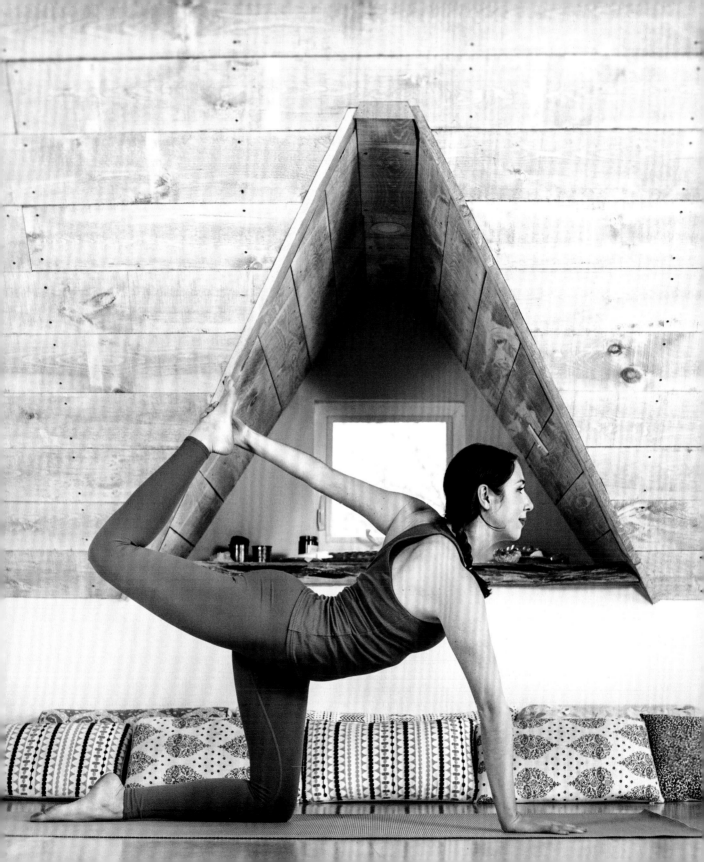

WINTER

*I wonder if the snow loves the trees and fields, that it kisses them so gently?
And then it covers them up snug, you know, with a white quilt; and
perhaps it says, "Go to sleep, darlings, till the summer comes again."*

—Lewis Carroll

The season of winter is an invitation to slow down and rest. It marks both the ending of a year as well as the beginning of a new one. During this time of transition, we can let go of the past and focus on what's to come.

With nature dormant all around us, we can make the most of this peaceful time by focusing on our innermost dreams and desires. The practices and tools in this chapter will support you in this work.

THEME: rest and dream

WORDS: slow, silence, self-care, intention setting, beginnings, wisdom, visualizing, planting seeds, withdrawing, potential, introspection, sleep, nourishing, spirituality, solitude, intuition

FEELINGS: curiosity, peace, calm

BEST TIME TO: Slow down and nourish yourself deeply. Do less, eat more, sleep more, relax, and practice self-care. Spend time going inward through journaling and meditation. Set intentions to get clear on what you want next. Visualize or make a vision board.

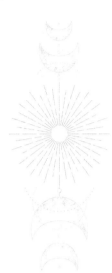

MORNING PRACTICE
Grounding Hatha

LEVEL: All Levels   **PROPS REQUIRED:** Block (optional)

This winter, begin each day with some gentle movement to wake up your body and focus your mind. Let's embrace the slow-paced nature of this season with a simple grounding sequence that will keep you close to the earth.

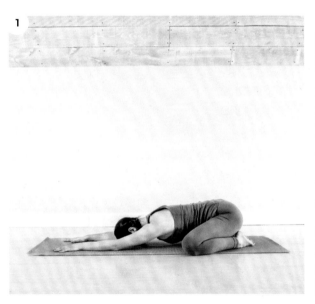

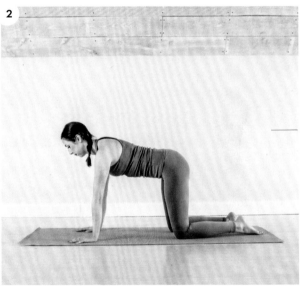

1. Extended Child's Pose (*Utthita Balasana*)
From your hands and knees, widen your knees to the edges of your mat and bring your big toes together to touch. Press your hips back toward your heels and extend your arms forward, gently lowering your forehead to the ground or to a block. Hold for ten breaths.

2. Table Top Pose (*Bharmanasana*)
Come back to your hands and knees and align your palms under your shoulders and your knees under your hips. Your spine should be straight with your abdominals engaged. Press into the floor with your fingertips and hold for five breaths.

Grounding happens when we connect to the earth physically, mentally, emotionally, and spiritually. Pay special attention to the parts of your body that are making contact with your mat and feel yourself supported by the ground beneath you.

As you practice, set your intention for the day ahead by choosing one word that captures how you want to feel today or what you want to focus on.

3

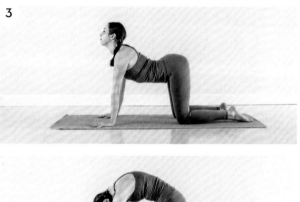
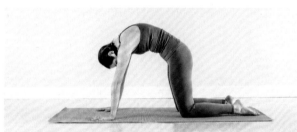

4

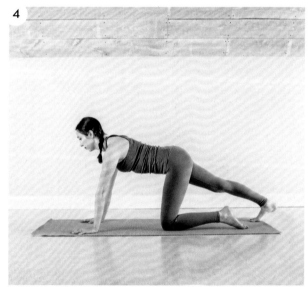

3. Cat/Cow Pose (*Marjaryasana/Bitilasana*)

From Table Top pose, inhale through your nose and arch your back as you stretch the front of your torso. Lift your gaze, drop your belly, and lift your tailbone up toward the sky.

Exhale through your nose and reverse this motion by rounding your back as you stretch along your spine. Drop your head, spread your shoulder blades wide, and let your tailbone be heavy.

Move in and out of these two poses for ten breath cycles.

4. Calf and Ankle Stretch

From Table Top pose, extend your right leg back and push the ball of your right foot into the mat as you reach your heel back at an angle. Hold for five breaths before repeating with the left leg.

Come back to Table Top pose.

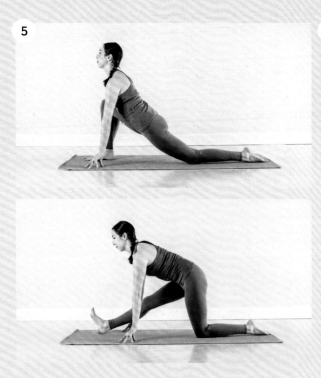

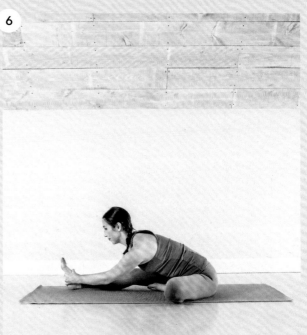

5. Equestrian Pose into Half Monkey Pose
(*Ashwa Sanchalanasana/Ardha Hanumanasana*)

Step your right foot forward between your palms and align your knee over your ankle. Melt your hips down toward the earth as you lift your chest and roll your shoulders back. Hold for five breaths.

Straighten your right leg and shift the weight of your hips back to stretch into your hamstrings. Flex your front foot and press down into your heel. Hold for five breaths.

Come back to Table Top pose and repeat both poses on the left side.

6. Head-to-Knee Pose (*Janu Sirsasana*)

Take a seat and extend your right leg out in front of you. Bend your left knee to rest the sole of your foot on the inside of your right thigh.

Inhale and reach your arms up over your head to lengthen your spine. As you exhale, hinge from your hips to fold over your right leg. Keep your back straight and bring your hands to each side of your right leg or hold on to your foot.

Hold for ten breaths before switching sides.

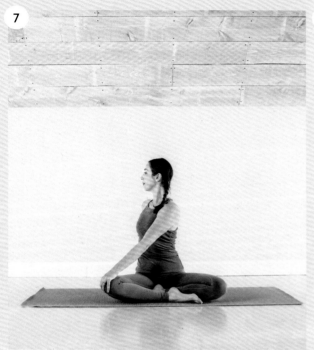

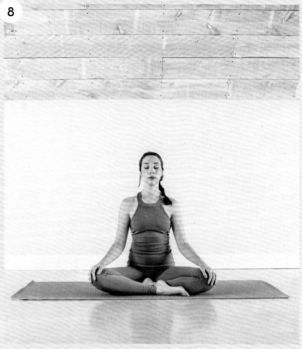

7. Easy Twist Pose (*Parivrtta Sukhasana*)

Sit cross-legged with your shoulders aligned over your hips. Bring your left palm to your right knee and your right hand behind you for support as you twist. Relax your shoulders and keep your spine straight. Hold for ten breaths before twisting to the other side.

8. Easy Pose (*Sukhasana*)

Finish this practice by sitting cross-legged on the floor or elevated on a block, resting your hands on your thighs with your palms facing down. Close your eyes, focus on the steady rhythm of your breath, and choose your intention for the day. Take ten breaths here.

Bring your palms together at your heart (*anjali mudra*), inhale through your nose, and chant om (*aum*) as you exhale.

EVENING MEDITATION

Five Senses Meditation

Our senses are a direct gateway to mindfulness. In this meditation, we'll utilize all five senses to practice mindfulness. Take five to fifteen minutes every evening to go through this simple meditation.

Begin by sitting in Easy pose (*Sukhasana*), cross-legged with your hips flat on the ground or elevated on a blanket or pillow. Place your hands in lotus (*padma*) mudra, the blossoming flower of the heart. Bring the base of your palms together to touch and open up your fingers, like a blossoming flower. Keep your thumbs and pinky fingers connected. This is a way for us to cultivate compassion for ourselves and others and get in touch with our inner abundance.

Take slow, steady breaths in and out through your nose.

Begin with the sense of sight. Rather than closing your eyes, look down into the center of your palms, gazing into the lotus flower blooming at your heart. Without judgment, observe the colors and the light as if you are seeing them for the very first time. Take ten to twenty deep breaths here.

Next, close your eyes and focus on your hearing. As you listen deeply, think about what sounds are present in your environment in the moment. Notice how near or far the sources of these sounds are. Focus on this for ten to twenty breaths.

Bring your attention to the sense of smell as the air naturally flows in and out through your nostrils. Notice if there are any scents that you can detect, without judging or labeling them. Stay with the sense of smell for ten to twenty breaths.

Focus now on your mouth and the sense of taste. Feel your tongue, the inside of your cheeks, and your teeth. You might swallow a few times to observe the sense of taste. Take ten to twenty breaths here.

Finally, bring your full awareness to the sense of touch. Feel the base of your palms together and the connection between your pinkies and thumbs. Notice the air around you, the feeling of your clothing, and the temperature of the room. Stay here for ten to twenty breaths.

Now bring all the senses together at once, increasing your attunement to what you can see, hear, smell, taste, and feel. Stay here for ten to twenty breaths before releasing the meditation.

When you're ready, release the mudra, open your eyes, and resume your evening.

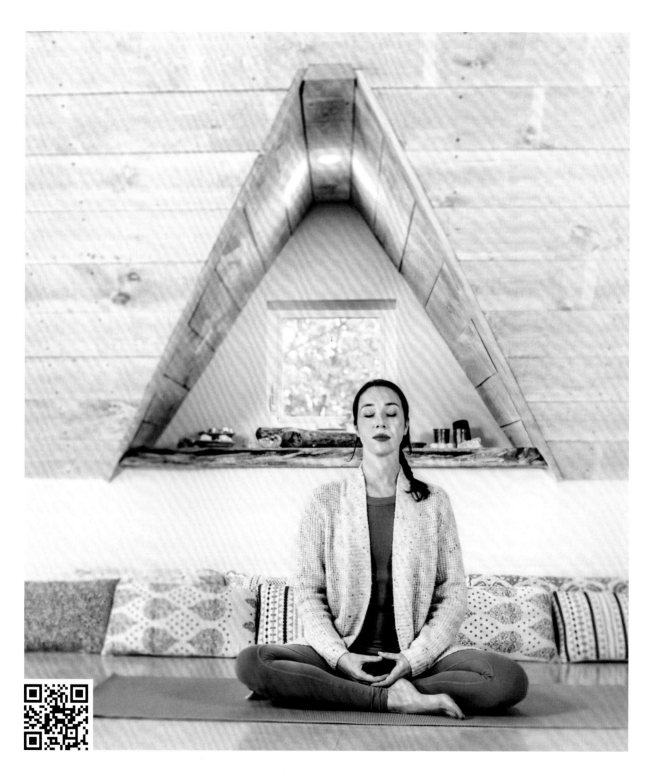

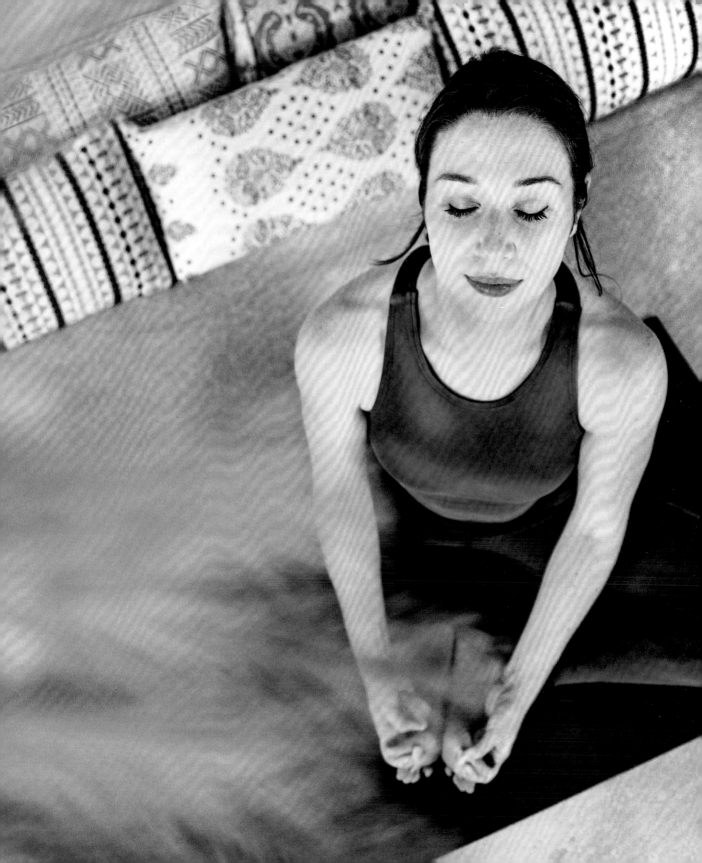

BREATHING EXERCISE

Ujjayi Pranayama

)))) ● ● ● ((((

Pranayama comes from the word *prana*, meaning life force, and *yama*, meaning constraint or regulation. *Ujjayi*, meaning breath of the conqueror or victorious breath, is a breath regulation technique that allows us to focus our awareness and calm the mind.

Ujjayi pranayama is performed by inhaling and exhaling through the nose with a slight constriction at the back of the throat. This constriction will cause a soft whispering sound like that of ocean waves or the sound you make when you fog up a mirror. The breath should be gentle and smooth, with the inhalations and exhalations equal in duration.

You can practice this technique by sitting comfortably in Easy pose (*Sukhasana*) cross-legged on your mat or a pillow. Close your eyes and bring awareness to your throat. With a slight constriction coming from the epiglottis, inhale slowly for a count of three to five. Maintain the constriction as you exhale for that same count of three to five. Continue for five to ten minutes. If you notice your mind drifting away, bring your awareness back to your breath. You can use the sound of your breath or the sensation of the breath as it travels through your nostrils as the anchor for your awareness.

This particular breathing technique can be used on its own or while doing each yoga practice and guided meditation found in this book.

AFFIRMATIONS

Affirmations are positive statements that can be used to uncover the parts of ourselves that have been cast away, rejected, or suppressed. They can also be used to motivate, inspire, and align our thoughts with our actions.

This winter, incorporate these affirmations into your morning or evening routine by repeating them internally or out loud. You might find it beneficial to journal right after doing this, in order to further integrate the process.

Our affirmations this season relate to self-care, rest, intention setting, and inner guidance.

1. I am unique, and it is my greatest strength.

2. I allow myself to slow down and enjoy life.

3. I trust the timing of my life.

4. I am safe, grounded, and stable.

5. My potential is endless.

6. I allow myself to dream big.

7. My thoughts, words, and actions are grounded in love.

8. Life supports me in every way.

9. It is safe for me to let go and relax.

10. I choose serenity and peace.

11. I see the bigger picture and trust my intuition.

12. I let go of all that no longer serves me.

13. I love myself deeply.

14. I take great care of myself.

15. I believe in my dreams and desires.

16. I am in the process of positive change.

17. Deep within me is an infinite source of love.

18. I feel at home in my body.

19. I am connected to my power center.

20. My journey is my own, and I claim it now.

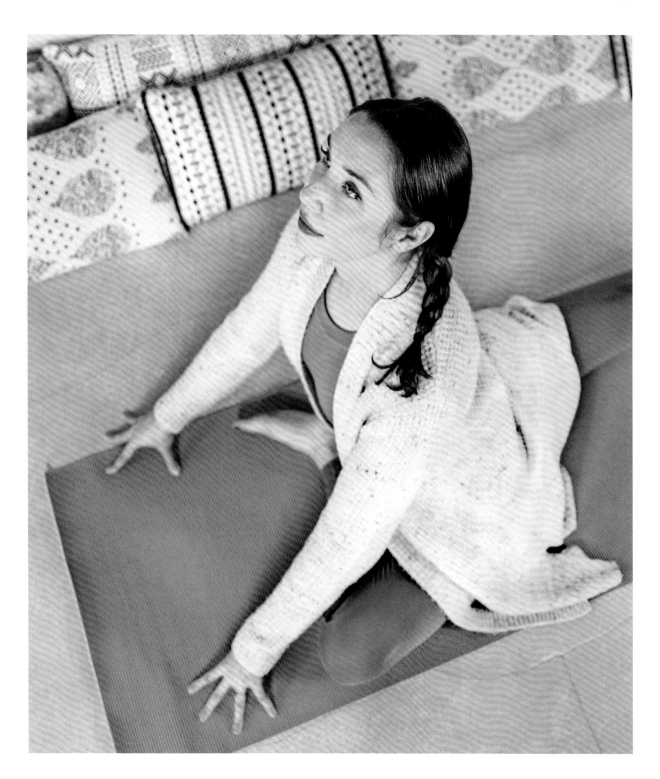

NEW MOON RITUAL

Vision Board

The new moon represents the vastness of potential, where all dreams and ideas are born. Now's the time to ask yourself the big questions: What do I want? What do I need? What is most important to me?

A great way to answer these questions is by making a vision board. Cut out images and words from magazines and paste them onto a board to solidify your vision for the next twelve months. During each new moon of the winter season, spend some time collecting images that represent your greatest vision of yourself.

Focus on what matters most to you and what you want to make a priority this year. If you're feeling stuck or overwhelmed, consider these areas of your life: health, relationships, spirituality, creativity, and lifestyle.

Make sure to only include elements of a vision that is truly yours, not what other people want for you or what you think you should want. Leave your board out somewhere you can see it every day, as a reminder of what is truly important to you.

FULL MOON RITUAL

Pampering Bath

I can't think of a better way to end a cold winter day than by drawing a warm, luscious bath. The purpose of a full moon bath ritual is to reconnect with yourself and recharge.

The key to a great bath is to incorporate the five senses and infuse meaning into the experience. For the sense of sight, use candles or ambient lighting; for smell, burn incense or light a scented candle that captures the mood; for taste, have dark chocolate, tea, or wine on hand; for hearing, use some of your favorite music or listen to a guided meditation; for touch, have some lotion or body oils ready for when you step out of the bath. You can also add two cups of Epsom salts to your bath to give your muscles an extra dose of TLC.

To take your experience further, you can incorporate the crystals, scents and oils, and playlist included in the winter listicle (pages 48–49).

Also, I recommend having a journal with you, as this can be a wonderful time to make a gratitude list or write out things you are ready to release. You might even be inspired to write some poetry or a song! Let your creativity and intuition be your guide.

LISTICLE

Tap into the energy of winter with the help of these resources. You'll find some inspirational books to set the tone for the season, a nourishing smoothie recipe, recommended reading, and more. Let yourself slow down and rest over the next few months.

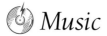 Music

"The Southern Sea" by Garth Stevenson
"Window" by The Album Leaf
"Ascent" by Josh Brill
"Let the Drummer Kick" by Citizen Cope
"Purnamadah" by Shantala
"Ink" by Coldplay
"Winter Birds" by Ray LaMontagne
"Gravity" by John Mayer
"Sound of Invisible Waters" by Deuter
"Flying" by Garth Stevenson
"Savasana II" by Gabriele Morgan

Books

The Desire Map by Danielle LaPorte
Meditations from the Mat by Rolf Gates
The Yoga Sutras of Patanjali by Sri Swami
     Satchidananda
Radical Acceptance by Tara Brach
Siddhartha by Hermann Hesse
The Yoga of the Nine Emotions by Peter
     Marchand

Crystals

AMETHYST: This crystal will help you tap into your imagination and give you a boost of inspiration. It has calming properties and can help improve the quality of your sleep and the vividness of your dreams.

LABRADORITE: Use this stone to tap into your creativity and deepest desires. When setting intentions, this crystal can help you see the bigger picture.

RED JASPER: Connected to the root (*Muladhara*) chakra, this stone helps you feel grounded and secure so that you can tap into your own inner power.

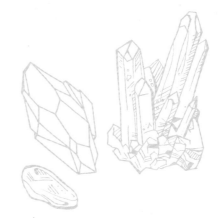

Scents & Oils

FRANKINCENSE: Use this oil as an accompaniment during meditation to facilitate spiritual connection. It is both uplifting and grounding.

EUCALYPTUS: Use this scent for a boost of energy and invigoration. It supports easy breathing and can lift your mood during the darkest winter days.

CLOVE: Use this scent for warmth and relaxation. Traditionally, this is thought to be a health booster, specifically for the respiratory and digestive systems.

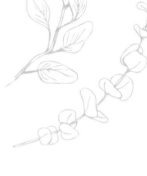

CHAKRA: Root (*Muladhara*)
ELEMENT: Earth
MOON PHASE: New Moon

CARDINAL DIRECTION: North
ZODIAC: Capricorn, Aquarius, Pisces

APPLE CINNAMON SMOOTHIE RECIPE

SERVES 1 TO 2

1 cup milk of choice
¼ cup oats
1 apple, core and seeds removed
1 banana
1 cup baby spinach
1 tablespoon almond butter
1 teaspoon cinnamon
¼ cup ice (optional)

Combine all ingredients in a blender. Blend until your desired consistency is reached. The almond butter can be substituted with peanut butter. If the smoothie is too thick, add an extra ½ cup of either milk or water.

YOGA SEQUENCE 1
Earth Element

LEVEL: All Levels   **PROPS REQUIRED:** None

Winter is associated with the element of earth, which is all about stability, wisdom, and inner strength. It is also connected to the root (*Muladhara*) chakra at the base of the spine. This all-levels grounding yoga sequence will help you deepen your own connection to the earth by working on foundational poses that target your feet and legs.

As you practice, visualize yourself as a great big tree. Imagine yourself rooting deep into the core of the earth from your tailbone and your feet while lengthening your spine and arms like the tallest branches. This is meant to be a strengthening and nourishing practice to help you feel supported, balanced, and stable.

1

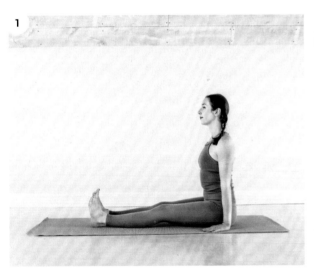

2

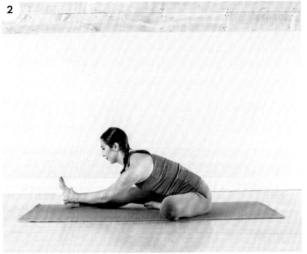

1. Staff Pose (*Dandasana*)

Sit with your legs extended out in front of you, pressing into your heels. Plant your palms firmly on the ground and straighten your spine. Hold for ten breaths, feeling your connection to the earth beneath you.

2. Head-to-Knee Pose (*Janu Sirsasana*)

Bend your left knee and rest your left foot on the inside of your right thigh. Inhale to lift your arms up and straighten your spine. Exhale to fold forward over your right thigh, tilting your pelvis forward. Hold for ten breaths before switching sides.

3

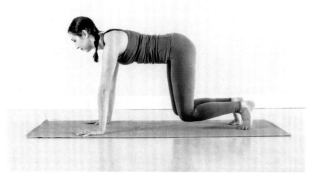

4

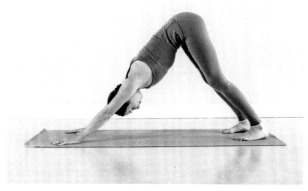

5

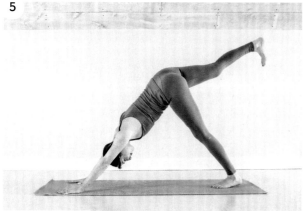

6

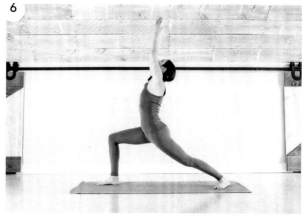

3. Table Top Pose Variation (*Bharmanasana*)

Come to all fours and spread your fingers wide. Curl your toes underneath you and lift your knees and shins to hover an inch off the ground. Engage your core and flatten your lower back. Hold for ten breaths.

4. Downward-Facing Dog Pose
(*Adho Mukha Svanasana*)

From all fours, walk your hands a few inches past your shoulders. Tuck your toes under and lift your hips up and back. Reach your chest toward your thighs and relax your neck. Hold for ten breaths.

5. Three-Legged Downward-Facing Dog Pose
(*Eka Pada Adho Mukha Svanasana*)

Lift your right leg up toward the sky, while keeping both hips parallel to the ground. Flex your right foot and push into your left heel, holding for five breaths.

6. Warrior 1 Pose (*Virabhadrasana 1*)

Step your right foot to the top of your mat and press your back heel down, placing your left foot at a 45-degree angle. Bend your front knee generously and reach your arms up overhead. Press your hands together and look up. Hold for five breaths.

7

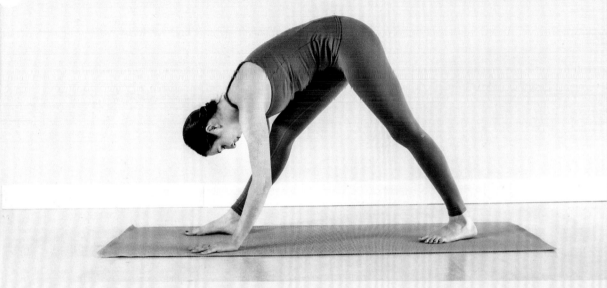

8

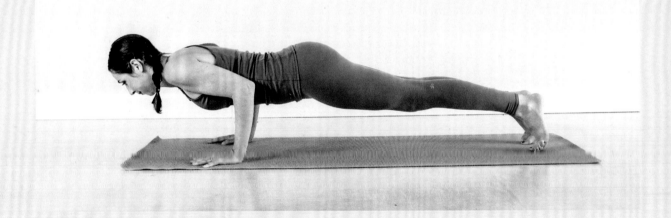

7. Pyramid Pose (*Parsvottanasana*)

Straighten your right leg and bring your back foot in a few inches. Hinge at your hips to fold down toward your right shin. Lengthen out of your low back and press evenly into both feet. Hold for ten breaths.

8. Vinyasa (see pages 20–21)

Bend your front knee and lower both hands down to step back into Plank pose. Flow from Plank to Four-Limbed Staff pose to Upward-Facing Dog and back to Downward-Facing Dog.

Repeat Three-Legged Downward-Facing Dog, Warrior 1, and Pyramid poses on the second side. Follow with a vinyasa.

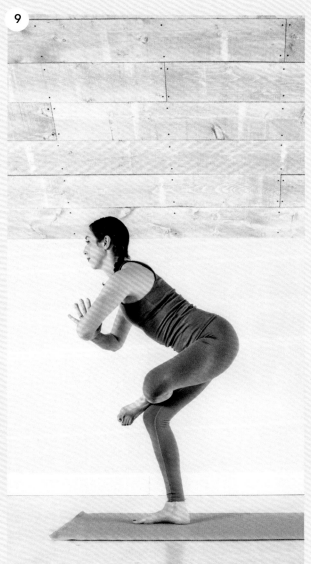

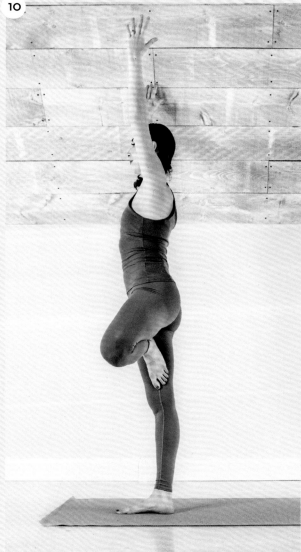

9. Standing Pigeon Pose
(*Tada Kapotasana*)
Come to standing and balance on your right leg by lifting up your left leg. Cross your left ankle over your right knee and bend into your supporting leg, shifting your hips back. Place your hands at your heart and hold for ten breaths. Repeat on the other side.

10. Tree Pose (*Vrksasana*)
Balance on your right leg and place your left foot on the inside of your right shin or right inner thigh. Engage your glutes to externally rotate your left hip. Press down into your right foot and extend your arms up overhead. Hold for ten breaths and repeat on the other side.

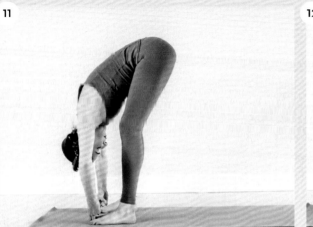

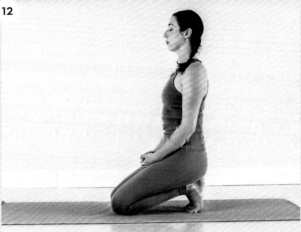

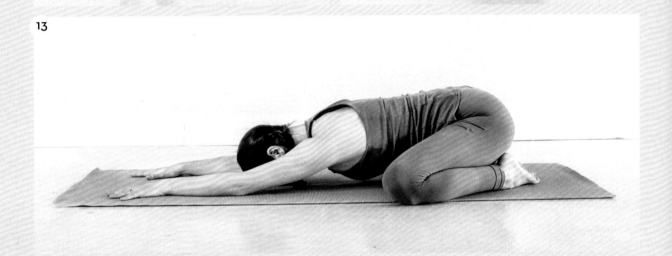

11. Big Toe Pose (*Padangusthasana*)

Start with your feet hip-width apart. Hinge forward at your hips to fold all the way down. Bend your knees if needed. Grab your big toes with your two index fingers and pull your elbows away from each other. Hold for ten breaths.

12. Thunderbolt Pose Variation (*Vajrasana*)

Come down to a kneeling position and tuck your toes underneath you to sit on your heels. Feel the stretch into the soles of your feet as you rest your hands on your lap. Hold for ten breaths.

13. Extended Child's Pose (*Utthita Balasana*)

From your hands and knees, widen your knees to the edges of your mat and bring your big toes together to touch. Press your hips back toward your heels and extend your arms forward, gently lowering your forehead to the ground or to a block. Hold for ten breaths.

14

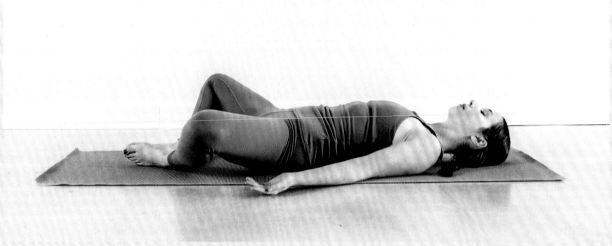

15

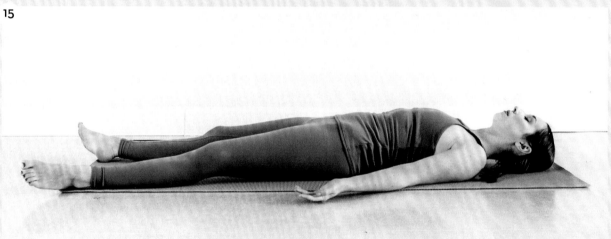

14. Reclined Butterfly Pose
(*Supta Baddha Konasana*)
Transition to your back. Bring the soles of your feet together to touch and let your knees fall open. Close your eyes and take ten deep breaths in and out through your nose.

15. Corpse Pose (*Savasana*)
Stretch your arms and legs out, turning your palms toward the sky. Relax your shoulders away from your ears, close your eyes, and breathe deeply. Stay for five minutes or longer.

YOGA SEQUENCE 2
Yoga for a Healthy Spine

LEVEL: All Levels   **PROPS REQUIRED:** None

I truly believe that proper posture is an essential component of good health. Whether you suffer from upper, middle, or lower back tension, this yoga sequence should bring you some relief and help you develop proper posture and alignment.

This is an accessible sequence for all levels that focuses on strength and flexibility. We will work on strengthening the muscles along your spine while also engaging your abdominal muscles. This sequence incorporates backbends, forward folds, twists, and side bends to stretch and release tension.

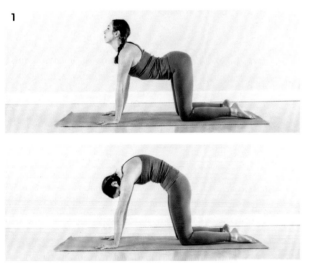

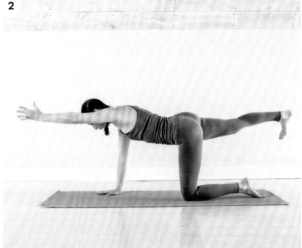

1. Cat/Cow Pose (*Marjaryasana/Bitilasana*)

From Table Top pose, inhale to arch your back and look up as you stretch the front of your torso. Exhale to reverse this motion by rounding your back and dropping your head to stretch along your spine. Move in and out of these two poses for ten breath cycles.

2. Balancing Table Top Pose
(*Dandayamana Bharmanasana*)

From Table Top pose, engage your abdominal muscles and flatten your lower back. Extend your right leg back behind you, parallel to the ground. Reach your left arm forward, bicep aligned with your ear. Hold here for ten breaths before switching sides.

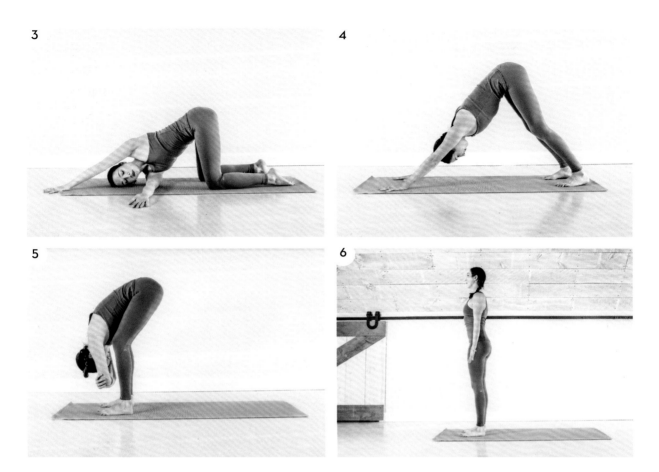

3. Thread the Needle Pose (*Parsva Balasana*)

From all fours, reach your right arm underneath you to lower your right shoulder and ear to the mat. Extend your left arm up over your head. Push your right arm and your left hand into the floor. Hold for five breaths before switching sides.

5. Standing Forward Bend Pose Variation (*Uttanasana*)

Walk your feet to the top of the mat so that your upper body dangles over your legs. Bend your knees as much as is comfortable. Relax your neck and hold on to your upper arms as you sway from side to side. Hold for ten breaths.

4. Downward-Facing Dog Pose (*Adho Mukha Svanasana*)

From Table Top pose, walk your hands a few inches past your shoulders. Tuck your toes under and lift your hips up and back. Reach your chest toward your thighs and press your heels toward the mat. Hold for ten breaths.

6. Mountain Pose (*Tadasana*)

Stand up tall at the top of your mat with your feet hip-width apart. Roll your shoulders back and turn your palms forward. Press into all four corners of both feet.

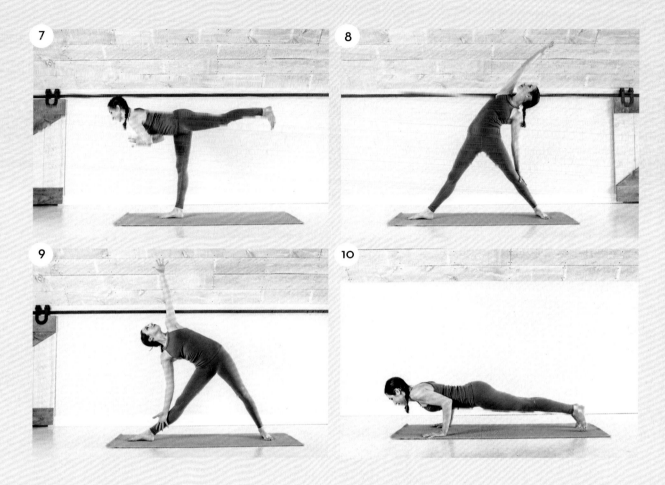

7. Warrior 3 Pose (*Virabhadrasana III*)

Lean on your right leg as you tilt forward and lift your left leg back behind you. Pull in your lower belly to protect your lower back until you are parallel to the ground. Bring your hands to your heart and hold for ten breaths.

8. Reverse Triangle Pose (*Viparita Trikonasana*)

Drop your left foot and align it with the short edge of your mat. Release your left arm down your left leg and reach your right arm up and back, coming into a side bend. Hold for five breaths.

9. Triangle Pose (*Trikonasana*)

Keep both legs straight and reach your hips back and chest forward. Extend your right arm forward and down to place your outer palm on your inner right shin. Extend your left arm up and hold for ten breaths.

10. Vinyasa (see pages 20–21)

Bend your front knee and lower both hands to step back into Plank pose. Flow from Plank to Four-Limbed Staff pose to Upward-Facing Dog and back to Downward-Facing Dog.

Repeat Warrior 3, Reverse Triangle, and Triangle poses on the second side. Follow with a vinyasa.

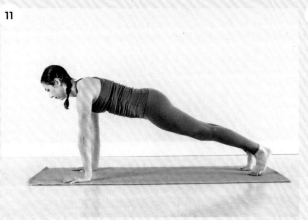

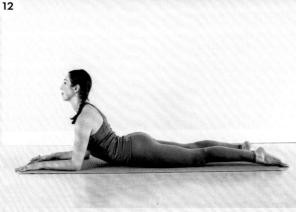

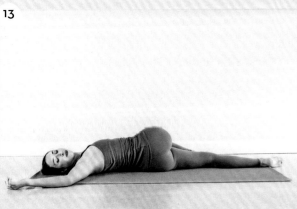

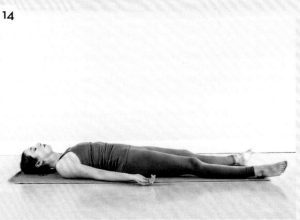

11. Plank Pose (*Kumbhakasana*)

Shift forward into Plank pose by aligning your shoulders over your wrists. Lower your knees to the mat to make this easier. Engage your abdominal muscles and hug your upper arms toward each other. Hold for ten breaths.

12. Sphinx Pose (*Salamba Bhujangasana*)

Lower to your belly and bring your forearms out in front of you. Lift your chest and press your pelvis into the ground. Roll your shoulders back and reach your heart forward. Hold for ten breaths.

13. Reclined Spinal Twist Pose
(*Supta Matsyendrasana*)

Flip over onto your back. Pull your right knee into your chest and extend your left leg straight. Cross your right thigh over your chest with the help of your left hand and extend your right arm out to the side. Gaze over your right shoulder and hold for ten breaths before switching sides.

14. Corpse Pose (*Savasana*)

Release the twist and stretch your arms and legs out, turning your palms toward the sky. Relax your shoulders away from your ears, close your eyes, and breathe deeply. Stay for five minutes or longer.

YOGA SEQUENCE 3
Yin Yoga for Deep Sleep

LEVEL: Beginner   **PROPS REQUIRED:** Block or bed pillow (optional)

If you're feeling the need to hibernate this season, this is the perfect yoga sequence for you! This yin yoga class will soothe your parasympathetic nervous system to help prepare you for a wonderful night's rest. If you have a difficult time falling or staying asleep, I recommend doing this practice right before bed.

This sequence is all about slow, simple movements to reduce stress and quiet down the mind. If you wanted to, you could even do this sequence in bed! Tuck yourself under the covers during Corpse pose and drift off to sleep.

1

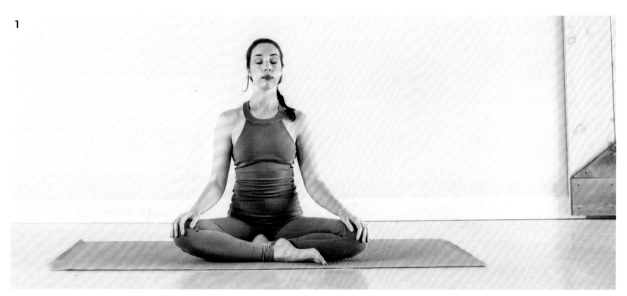

1. Seated Meditation
Begin by sitting comfortably with your shoulders stacked over your hips. Rest your palms on your lap and close your eyes. Breathe slowly for a few minutes as you relax each muscle of your body from head to toe.

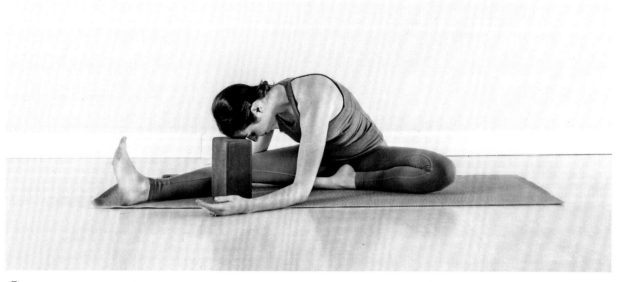

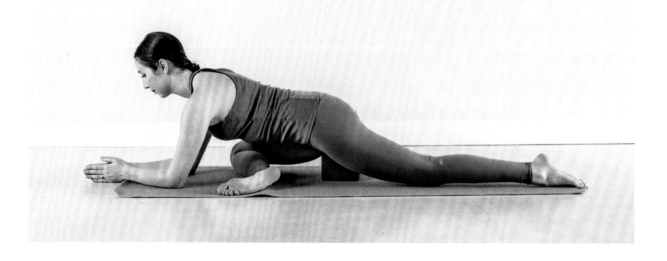

2. Half Butterfly Pose

Extend your right leg out to the side and bring your left foot to your inner right thigh. Walk your hands forward as you fold all the way down. You can use a block or pillow under your head for more support. Hold for three to five minutes before coming out and switching sides.

3. Swan Pose

Move to your hands and knees and place your right knee behind your right wrist. Stretch your back leg out behind you. You can place a block or pillow under your hips to level your pelvis. Come down to your forearms or lower all the way down for more sensation. Hold for three to five minutes.

4

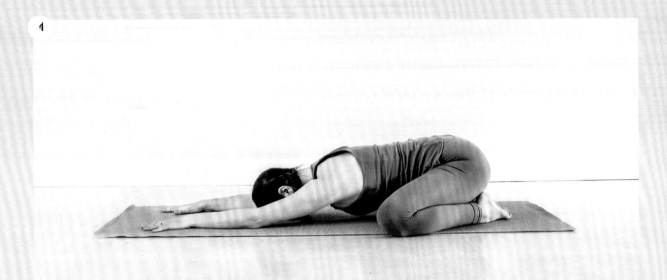

5

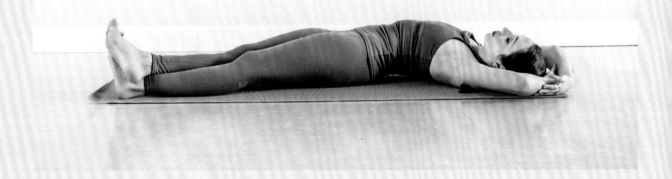

4. Child's Pose

Come out of Swan pose and touch your big toes together with your knees wide apart. Press your hips back toward your heels and walk your hands forward to melt your chest and forehead down. Hold here for three to five minutes.

Repeat Swan pose on the second side.

5. Banana Pose

Lie down on your back and bring your hips to the right and your shoulders and legs to the left, creating a banana shape with your body. Reach your arms up overhead to hold on to your elbows and cross your right ankle over your left. Press your right hip down and hold for three to five minutes before repeating on the other side.

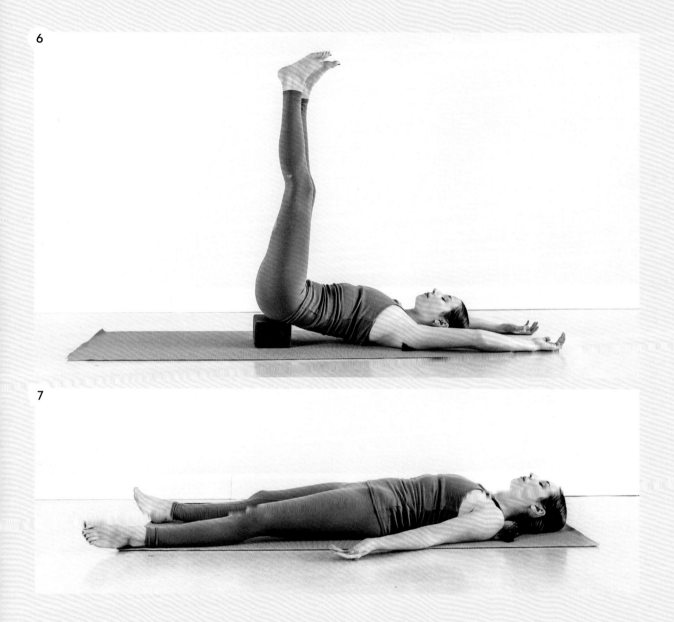

6. Waterfall Pose

Extend your legs straight up toward the sky. If you'd like more support, you can choose to rest your heels against the wall. You might also want to prop a pillow or block under your hips. Reach your arms up overhead and hold for three to five minutes.

7. Corpse Pose

Lower your legs and remove your props if you used any. If you're in bed, you can choose to get under the covers. Extend your legs out one at a time and bring your arms down by your sides. Close your eyes and breathe deeply, letting yourself drift off to sleep.

YOGA SEQUENCE 4
Yoga for Focus & Clarity

LEVEL: Intermediate   **PROPS REQUIRED:** None

Doing yoga is a great way to sharpen your mind. If you're feeling lethargic, this sequence will help clear away brain fog. This practice mainly uses balancing and asymmetrical poses, as they require focus and concentration to perform. We'll also be employing the nadi shodhana breathing technique (page 77) to facilitate inner equilibrium. By the end of the practice, you should feel alert and clear.

It's important to keep in mind that our ability to maintain balance in poses can change dramatically from day to day. If you find that you're struggling or wobbly, stay patient with yourself and don't take it too seriously!

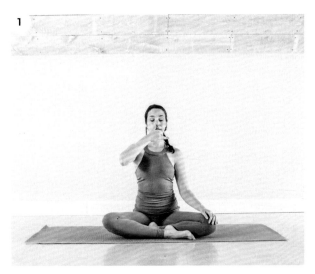

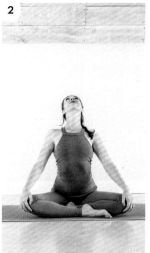

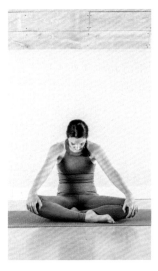

1. Alternate Nostril Breath (*Nadi Shodhana*) (see page 77)
Sit comfortably and use your right hand to perform ten rounds of nadi shodhana

2. Seated Cat/Cow Pose
(*Upavistha Marjaryasana/Bitilasana*)
Place your hands on your knees and inhale to arch your back and squeeze your shoulder blades together. Reverse this motion as you exhale and round your spine. Repeat these two poses for ten breath cycles.

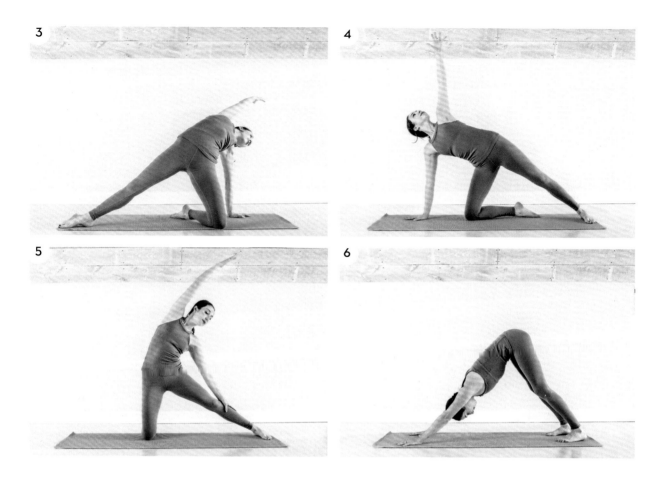

3. Baby Wild Thing Pose (*Camatkarasana*)

Extend your right leg out to the side and bring your left foot to your groin. Place your left hand back behind you and push into the floor to lift your hips up. Reach your right arm up and back. Hold for five breaths before switching sides.

5. Gate Pose (*Parighasana*)

Lower your left foot to the mat and use core strength to lift your chest up. Stack your shoulders over your hips and reach your right arm up and over, coming into a side bend. Rest your left hand on your left leg. Hold for five breaths.

Repeat Side Plank Variation and Gate pose on the second side.

4. Side Plank Pose Variation (*Vasisthasana*)

Move to your hands and knees and straighten your left leg back behind you. Roll to the inside of your left foot and reach your left arm up. Hold here or make this more challenging by lifting your left leg off the mat at hip level. Hold for ten breaths.

6. Downward-Facing Dog Pose
(*Adho Mukha Svanasana*)

From all fours, walk your hands a few inches past your shoulders. Tuck your toes under and lift your hips up and back. Reach your chest toward your thighs and relax your neck. Hold for ten breaths.

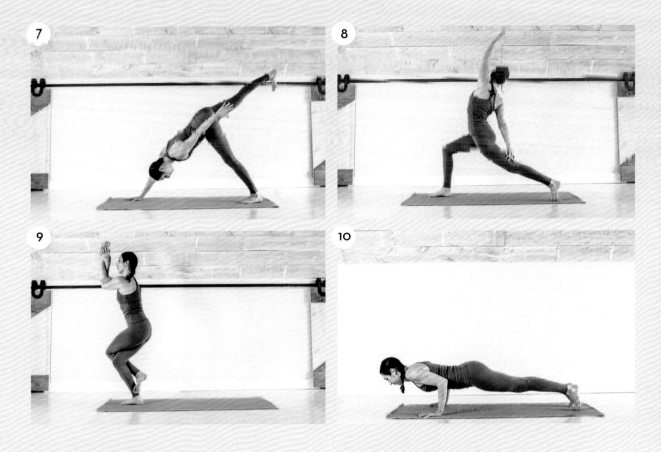

7. Two-Legged Downward-Facing Dog Pose Variation (*Dwi Pada Adho Mukha Svanasana*)

Lift your right leg up toward the sky, keeping your hips level with one another and parallel to the ground. Come up onto your left fingertips and slowly lift and reach your left arm back, bringing it in line with your right leg. Hold for ten breaths.

9. Eagle Pose (*Garudasana*)

From your high lunge, step to the top of your mat. Balance on your right leg and cross your left thigh over, hooking your left foot behind your right calf. Bend your elbows and wrap your left arm under your right and wrap your wrists. Bend deeply into your supporting leg and hold for ten breaths.

8. Exalted Crescent High Lunge Pose (*Parivrtta Viparita Ashta Chandrasana*)

Step your right foot forward to the top of your mat and lift up your chest. Twist to the right as you place your right hand on your upper left thigh. Extend your left arm up and over to deepen the side bend. Hold for ten breaths.

10. Vinyasa (see pages 20–21)

Release Eagle pose and fold down to place both palms down. Step your feet back into Plank pose. Flow from Plank to Four-Limbed Staff pose to Upward-Facing Dog and back to Downward-Facing Dog.

Repeat the Two-Legged Downward-Facing Dog Variation, Exalted Crescent High Lunge and Eagle pose on the second side. Add a vinyasa.

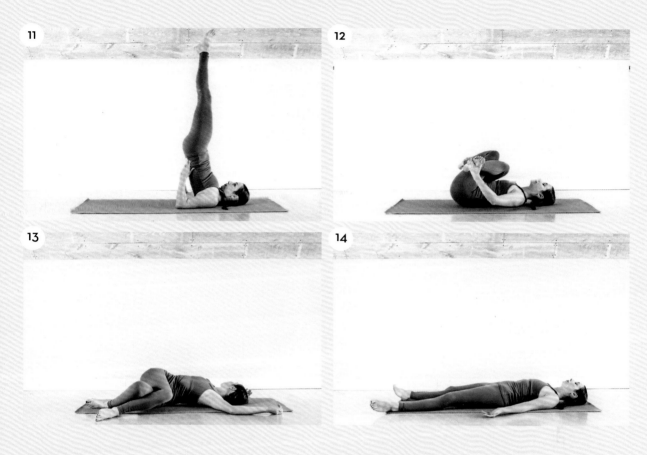

11. Shoulderstand Pose (*Sarvangasana*)

Lower all the way down onto your back. Bring your knees into your chest to lift your hips off the ground. Place your hands to your lower back as you straighten your legs up toward the sky. Push down into your shoulders and reach up through your toes. Hold for ten breaths.

12. Reclined Cow Face Pose (*Supta Gomukhasana*)

Lower your legs down and cross your right thigh over your left. Use your hands to pull your feet away from one another while drawing your thighs in closer to your chest. Relax your head and shoulders on the mat. Hold here for ten breaths.

13. Reclined Eagle Twist Pose

(*Supta Parivrtta Garudasana*)

Keep the cross of your legs as you drop both knees over to the left. Open your arms out into a cactus shape and gaze over your right shoulder. Hold for ten breaths.

Come back through to the center and repeat Reclined Cow Face pose and Reclined Eagle Twist pose on the other side.

14. Corpse Pose (*Savasana*)

Release the twist and extend your arms and legs out, turning your palms toward the sky. Soften your shoulders away from your ears, close your eyes, and breathe deeply. Stay for five minutes or longer.

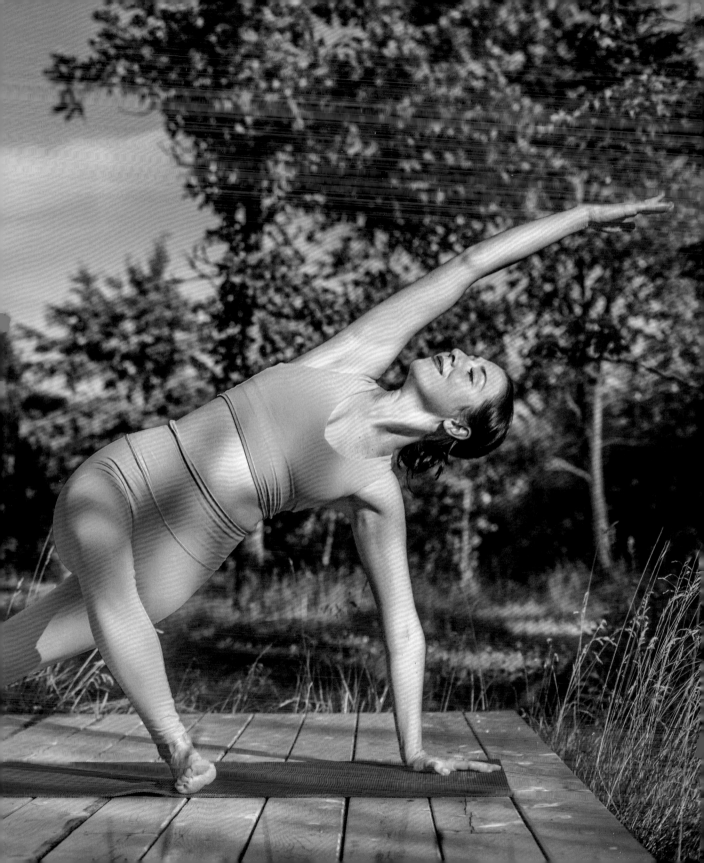

SPRING

It is spring again. The earth is like a child that knows poems by heart.

—Rainer Maria Rilke

The energy of spring is all about potential! Now's the time to move out into the world with a fresh new perspective as we embrace the return of longer and sunnier days. The practices in this section will help you tap into the power of this season.

Watch the intentions you set in winter begin to unfold and manifest in your life. The yoga practices, meditations, breathing exercises, affirmations, and lunar rituals will support you on this journey in spring.

THEME: take action

WORDS: play, begin, intuit, risk, plan, energy, act, balance, clarity, courage, renewal, new adventures

FEELINGS: joy, optimism, playfulness

BEST TIME TO: Take concrete action. Plan your next steps, start over, and launch. Try something new—maybe begin a new routine or take a risk. Acknowledge inner resistance and face your shadow. Confront old patterns and negative beliefs.

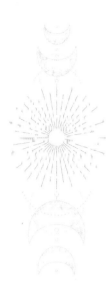

MORNING PRACTICE
Energy Boosting Flow

LEVEL: All Levels   **PROPS REQUIRED:** Block (optional)

This season's morning practice focuses primarily on spinal rotation and lateral flexion, also known as twists and side bends. This combination of poses is a wonderful way to activate your digestive system and get a boost of energy.

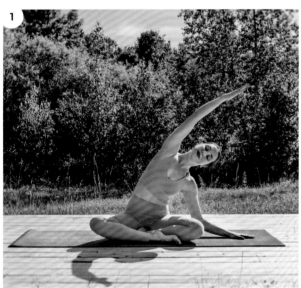

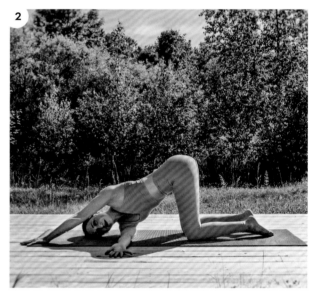

1. Seated Side Bend Pose (*Parsva Sukhasana*)

Sit comfortably in a cross-legged position with your spine tall and your shoulders down. Inhale to reach your right arm up and over into a side bend. Relax your neck and stay here for five breaths before switching to the other side.

2. Thread the Needle Pose (*Parsva Balasana*)

Come to a Table Top position on all fours. Reach your right arm underneath you toward the left side of your mat with your palm facing up. Lower your right shoulder and ear to the mat and extend your left arm up overhead. Push your right arm and your left hand into the floor. Hold for five breaths before switching sides.

We are shaking off the stagnant energy of winter and waking up from within, ready to embrace the day ahead! As you move through this sequence, emphasize the easy flow of your breath. You might choose to use ujjayi pranayama (see page 43) throughout to focus your awareness. Use your time on the mat to set your intention for the day ahead.

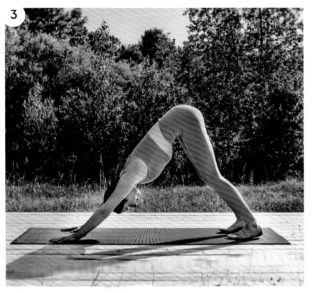

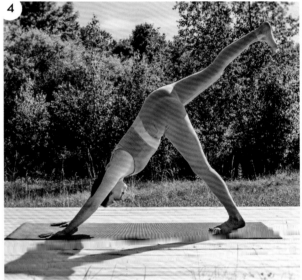

3. Downward-Facing Dog Pose
(*Adho Mukha Svanasana*)
From Table Top pose, walk your hands a few inches past your shoulders. Tuck your toes under and lift your hips up and back. Bend your knees if needed. Reach your chest toward your thighs and relax your neck. Hold for ten breaths.

4. Three-Legged Downward-Facing Dog Pose
(*Eka Pada Adho Mukha Svanasana*)
Lift your right leg up toward the sky, keeping both hips at the same height and parallel to the ground. Flex your right foot and push into your left heel, holding for five breaths.

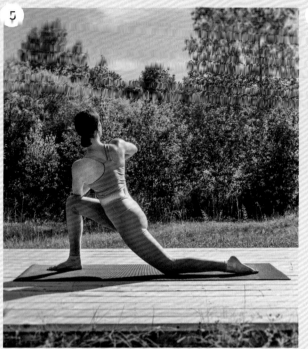

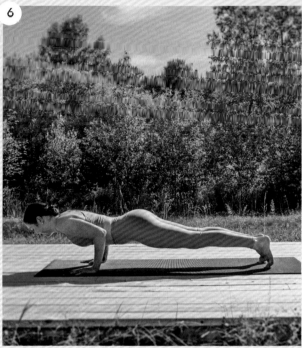

5. Low Lunge Twist Pose (*Parivrtta Anjaneyasana*)
Step that right foot through in between your palms, aligning your knee over your ankle. Lower your back knee to the earth. Bring your hands together in prayer and place your left elbow on your right thigh to initiate the twist. Hold for five breaths.

6. Vinyasa (see pages 20–21)
Release the Low Lunge Twist and place both palms down to step your feet back into Plank pose. Flow from Plank to Four-Limbed Staff pose to Upward-Facing Dog and back to Downward-Facing Dog.

Repeat Three-Legged Downward-Facing Dog and Low Lunge Twist poses on the second side. Follow with a vinyasa.

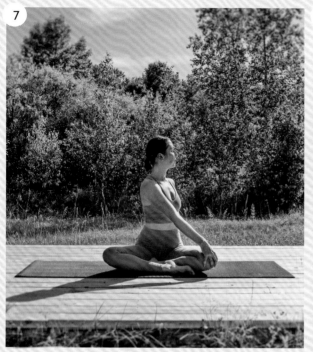

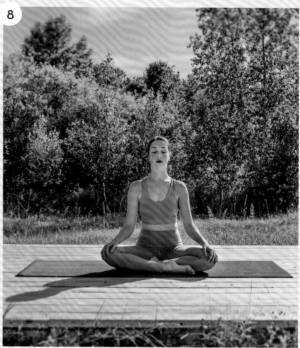

7. Easy Twist Pose (*Parivrtta Sukhasana*)

Come to a cross-legged sitting position. Place your right hand on your left knee and your left hand behind you for support. Lengthen your spine as you inhale and twist over to the left as you exhale, gazing over your left shoulder. Hold for five breaths before switching sides.

8. Easy Pose (*Sukhasana*)

Finish this practice by sitting cross-legged on the floor or elevated on a block, resting your hands on your thighs. Close your eyes, focus on the steady rhythm of your breath, and choose your intention for the day. Take ten breaths here.

Bring your palms together at your heart (*añjali mudra*), inhale through your nose, and chant om (aum) as you exhale.

EVENING MEDITATION

Metta Meditation

This season's evening meditation comes from the Buddhist practice of *Metta*, or loving kindness.

The practice involves directing loving kindness toward yourself, someone you love, someone you are neutral toward, and finally, someone you have difficulty with. It is a powerful meditation that teaches us the true essence of an open heart.

To begin, sit comfortably with your spine straight and your eyes closed. Take a few moments to breathe and feel the tension of the day melt away.

Focus on yourself first. Visualize yourself in this very moment and connect with your own worthiness, beauty, and essence. As you sit and breathe, internally repeat the following Metta phrases: "May I be happy. May I be healthy. May I be safe. May I be at ease." Sit with this for a few minutes before moving on.

Focus now on someone you love, maybe a friend who is dear to you. Visualize them sitting in front of you, and see them in their own worthiness, beauty, and essence. Allow your feelings of love for them to overflow. Internally bless them with the Metta phrases: "May you be happy. May you be healthy. May you be safe. May you be at ease." Sit with this for a few minutes before moving on.

Focus now on someone you feel neutral toward. It could be someone you don't know very well, such as an acquaintance, a neighbor, or a coworker. Just like you, this person desires happiness, safety, and health. Visualize them sitting in front of you and send them loving kindness with the Metta phrases: "May you be happy. May you be healthy. May you be safe. May you be at ease." Sit with this for a few minutes before moving on.

Finally, focus on someone you have difficulty with. This can be someone who irritates you or someone you disagree with. Even though you may not like them, visualize them in front of you and open your heart to their own worthiness and desire for health and happiness. As you sit and breathe, internally repeat the following Metta phrases: "May you be happy. May you be healthy. May you be safe. May you be at ease." Sit with this for a few minutes.

Although you might not fully believe in the blessings right now, with practice, it becomes easier to wish loving kindness to all living beings, including those you don't see eye to eye with.

Once you are ready to close the meditation, bring your palms to your heart and chant om (aum) one time. Slowly open your eyes and resume your evening with an open heart.

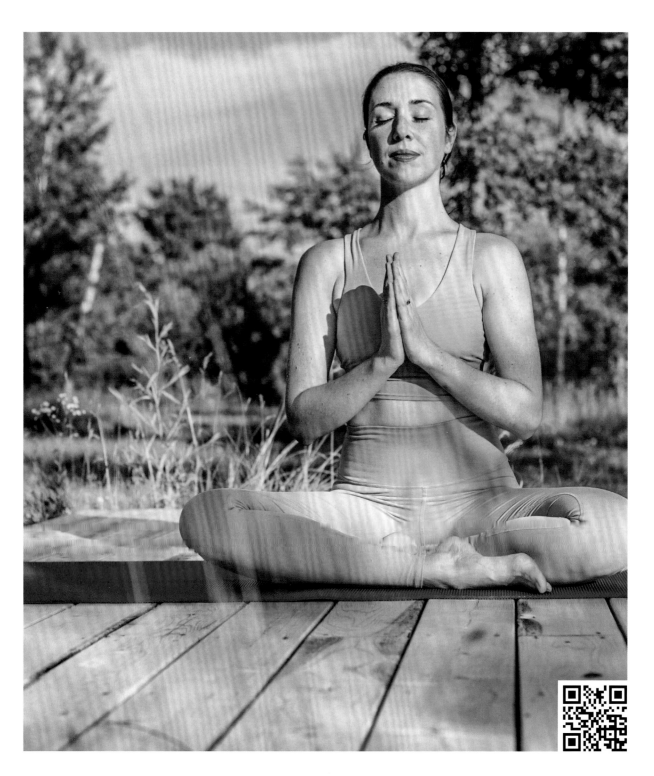

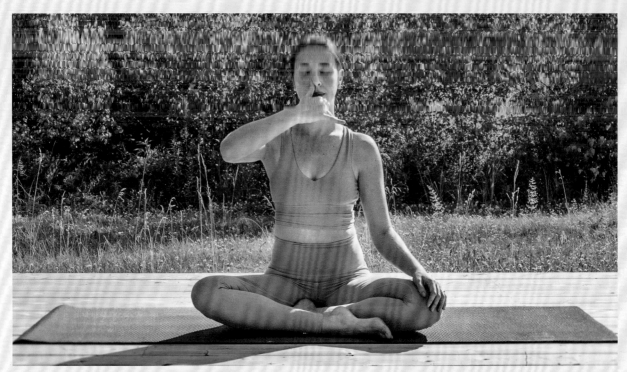

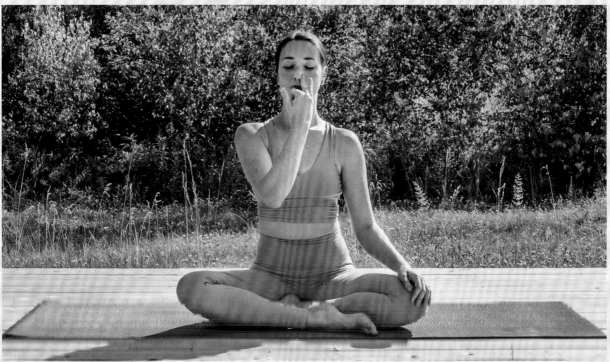

BREATHING EXERCISE

Nadi Shodhana

If you ever feel overwhelmed or overstimulated, *nadi shodhana* is an excellent pranayama technique to employ. This exercise, also known as alternate nostril breathing, helps bring balance and equilibrium to the nervous system.

It is ideally performed before or after your morning yoga practice, but it is suitable at any other time of the day.

Begin by sitting comfortably and placing your left hand on your thigh. Lift your right hand and curl your index and middle fingers into your palm. You'll be using your right thumb and ring finger for this practice.

1. *Use your right thumb to seal your right nostril, then inhale through your left nostril for a count of four, five, or six. Don't strain, the breath should be comfortable.*

2. *Use your right ring finger to close your left nostril, release your thumb from your right nostril and exhale for a count of four, five, or six.*

3. *Inhale through your right nostril for another count of four, five, or six.*

4. *Close your right nostril with your thumb, release your right ring finger from your left nostril, and exhale for a count of four, five, or six.*

Those four steps count as one round of nadi shodhana. You can repeat for five to ten rounds as is appropriate and comfortable to you. When you're done, take a few deep breaths through both nostrils and observe the effects of your practice.

AFFIRMATIONS

This season's positive affirmations relate to initiation, trust in ourselves, and confidence. Just like the flowers that blossom in spring, this is also our time to awaken and come alive!

Incorporate these affirmations into your morning or evening routine by repeating them internally or out loud. Observe what they awaken within you. Notice what you feel in your body, what thoughts or memories come up for you, and what beliefs you might associate with each affirmation. You might find it beneficial to journal right after doing this to further integrate the process.

1. *My day begins and ends with gratitude.*
2. *I adapt to change easily and effortlessly.*
3. *I am filled with creative energy.*
4. *I'm doing my best, and that's enough.*
5. *I allow abundance into my life.*
6. *I am a magnet for miracles.*
7. *I easily balance work and play.*
8. *I am a force of good in the world.*
9. *My priorities are crystal clear.*
10. *I dedicate time each day to taking care of myself.*
11. *I attract the right circumstances at the right time*
12. *I have all of the answers within me.*
13. *Good things are coming my way, and I'm ready for them.*
14. *I have the power to create change.*
15. *I'm open to new and exciting opportunities.*
16. *I give myself permission to heal.*
17. *My mind, body, and spirit are in perfect harmony.*
18. *My confidence inspires others.*
19. *I celebrate my inner and outer beauty.*
20. *I'm ready to take the next step.*

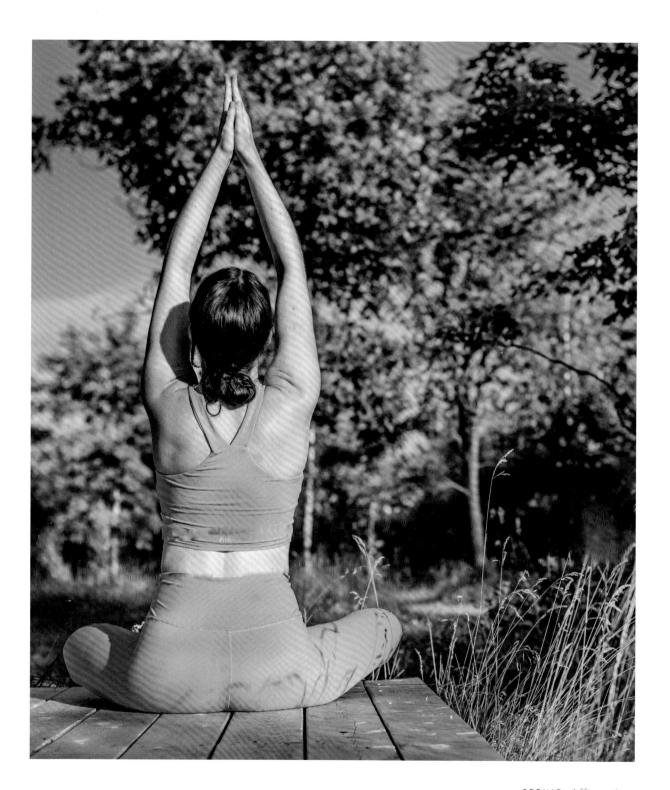

NEW MOON RITUAL

Planting Intentions

The new moon is a time to dream and set intentions. Use the energy of spring to take your intention and plant it in the soil as an act of commitment to your deepest wishes and desires.

You'll need a small pot, some soil, a piece of paper, a pen, and a seed. I like to use dwarf sunflower seeds, because they are easy to find and grow, but you can go with whatever you prefer.

Carve out some time during the new moon to meditate and choose your intention for the month. When you're ready, write your intention down on a piece of paper and place it inside your pot. Fill it with soil and plant your seed, visualizing your intention coming to life as you do this.

You'll need to give this little plant love and attention throughout the month. Nourish the seedling with some moon water (page 81) and nurture this plant and your intention as you watch it grow. If you'd like, adorn this little pot with crystals that support the season or your intention (page 82). Make this your own and watch your intentions come to life!

FULL MOON RITUAL

Moon Water

Looking to add a bit of magic to your life? Try moon water! This is a simple way to connect with lunar energy throughout the month. Symbolically, the moon represents the feminine, the subconscious, and the intuitive parts of ourselves that wax and wane in a cyclical nature. The full moon is associated with healing, gratitude, celebration, and compassion.

When the moon is full, fill a clear container of your choice, such as a mason jar, with fresh, drinkable water. You can add water-safe crystals to your container, such as rose quartz, moonstone, clear quartz, amethyst, citrine, or aventurine. Leave the container in direct moonlight overnight, either outdoors or indoors on a windowsill. Take a few minutes to recall the intention you set at the time of the new moon, and imagine this intention pouring into the water with the moonbeams amplifying this vision.

This water is meant to support your intention. Use it to water your plants or brew tea, add it to your bath, or simply drink it as is and enjoy!

LISTICLE

Enjoy the following recommended resources to feel your best this spring! You'll find a great playlist that can accompany your yoga practices, some recommended reading for inspiration, and other tools to help you connect to the energy of the season.

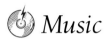 ## Music

"Chimes of Peace" by Adam Lees
"As I Wake in the Morning" by Alexia Chellun
"In My Life" by Jake Shimabukuro
"The Mountain" by Trevor Hall
"Dreams" by Fleetwood Mac
"Green & Gold" by Lianne La Havas
"Light Me Up" by DJ Drez featuring
    Marti Nikko
"Thinkin Bout You" by Frank Ocean
"Fly Like an Eagle" by Steve Miller Band
"I Am Light" by India.Arie
"Pachamama" by Beautiful Chorus
"Horizon" by Garth Stevenson
"Peace" by Lisbeth Scott

 ## Books

Living Your Yoga by Judith Hanson Lasater
Being Mortal by Atul Gawande
Embrace Yoga's Roots by Susanna Barkataki
A Return to Love by Marianne Williamson
The Untethered Soul by Michael A. Singer
Tantra Illuminated by Christopher Wallis

 ## Crystals

CARNELIAN: This stone is said to boost creativity and vitality. It offers healing energy and gives us the courage to try something new.

AVENTURINE: Think of this as your good-luck charm! As you move forward with your dreams and goals, aventurine supports you in forward positive action. Use this stone when taking risks.

ROSE QUARTZ: This stone is closely related to the heart (*Anahata*) chakra. It helps us connect to love and compassion and helps us have an open heart. The soft pink color is also reminiscent of cherry blossoms and other spring flowers.

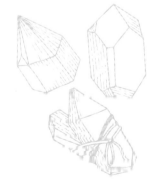

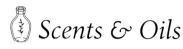

Scents & Oils

NEROLI: Use this floral scent to evoke peaceful and soothing energy.

PEPPERMINT: Get a boost of energy and clear away brain fog with the invigorating peppermint scent.

GRAPEFRUIT: Refresh your senses and gain mental clarity with this citrus scent.

CHAKRA: Heart (*Anahata*)

ELEMENT: Air

MOON PHASE: Waxing Moon

CARDINAL DIRECTION: East

ZODIAC: Aries, Taurus, Gemini

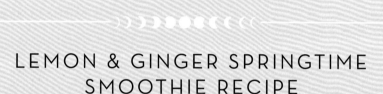

LEMON & GINGER SPRINGTIME SMOOTHIE RECIPE

SERVES 1 TO 2

1 cup arugula

1 cup baby spinach

1 cup water

1 apple, core and seeds removed

1 cup mango (fresh or frozen)

½ lemon, juiced

1 tablespoon fresh minced ginger (to taste)

½ teaspoon turmeric

¼ cup ice (optional)

Combine all ingredients in a blender and add ice if desired. Blend until your desired consistency is reached. You can make it thicker by adding half an avocado or a few tablespoons of Greek yogurt. Or make it sweeter by adding a tablespoon or two of honey.

YOGA SEQUENCE 1
Air Element

EVEL: Intermediate   **PROPS REQUIRED:** Strap (optional)

Spring is associated with the element of air, which corresponds to the heart (*Anahata*) chakra. Air is all about conscious breathing and deep connection to ourselves and others.

Physically, this flow will focus on the space of the heart and lungs through backbends, chest openers, and pranayama. When we tap into the element of air, we open ourselves up to the world emotionally. We allow ourselves to connect to our own life force and to all other living beings in the world.

This is a beautiful practice to do when you feel disconnected or lonely. It will remind you that no matter how far away your friends and family may be, they are all breathing the same air.

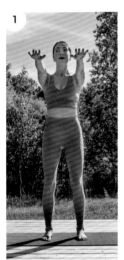 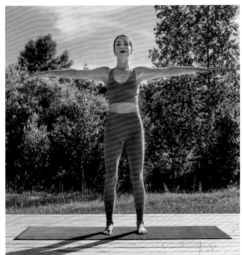 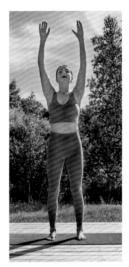 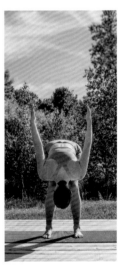

1. Breath of Joy

This is a four-part breathing sequence composed of three short inhales and one big exhale. Begin standing with your feet hip-width apart. Inhale through your nose and lift your arms out in front of you parallel to the ground. Inhale again to swing your arms down and up to your sides at shoulder height. Inhale one more time to swing your arms down and up overhead. Exhale out of your mouth as you fold forward over your thighs and swing your arms back. Repeat for ten rounds.

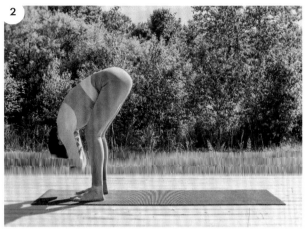

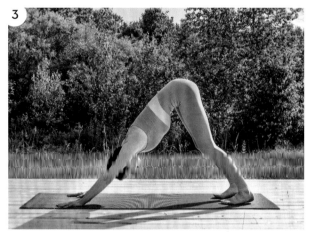

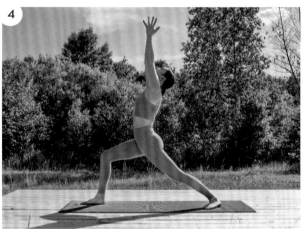

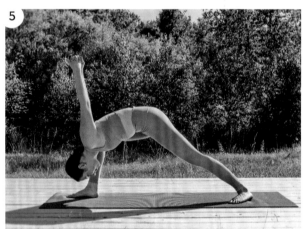

2. Standing Forward Bend Pose Variation (*Uttanasana*)

Hinge at your hips to fold forward, bending your knees as needed for comfort. Hold on to your upper arms as you dangle, gently rocking from side to side. Stay here for five breaths.

4. Warrior 1 Pose (*Virabhadrasana I*)

Step your right foot to the top of your mat and press your back heel down, placing your left foot at a 45-degree angle. Bend your front knee generously and reach your arms up overhead. Press your hands together and look up. Hold for five breaths.

3. Downward-Facing Dog Pose (*Adho Mukha Svanasana*)

Plant your palms on the mat and walk your feet back into Downward-Facing Dog pose. Spread your fingertips wide and reach your hips up and back. Hold for ten breaths.

5. Humble Warrior Pose (*Baddha Virabhadrasana*)

Clasp your hands behind your back or use a strap. Dive down toward the mat to the inside of your right thigh and reach your knuckles up and over. Hold for five breaths.

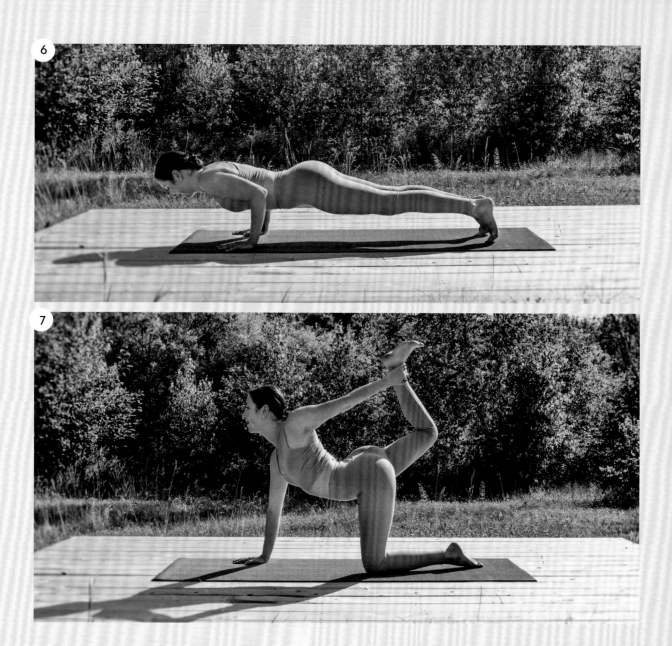

6. Vinyasa (see pages 20–21)

Release the previous pose and flow through a vinyasa.

Repeat Warrior 1 and Humble Warrior poses on the second side. Follow with a vinyasa.

7. One-Handed Tiger Pose (*Eka Hasta Vyaghrasana*)

Come down onto all fours. Arch your back and look up as you lift your right leg without externally rotating your thigh. Reach back with your left hand to hold your right ankle or use a strap. Hold for five breaths and repeat on the second side.

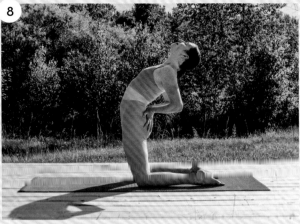

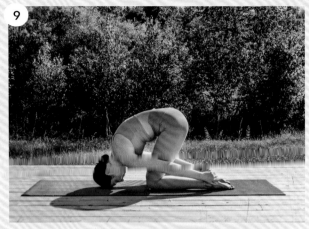

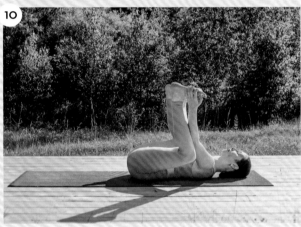

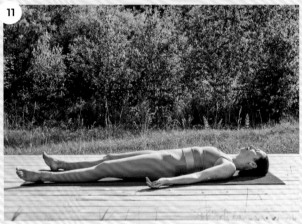

8. Camel Pose (*Ustrasana*)

Lift up onto your shins and align your pelvis over your knees. Place your hands behind your lower back and squeeze your shoulder blades together. Keep your hands there as you lift up from your chest and arch back into your backbend. Hold for ten breaths.

9. Rabbit Pose (*Sasangasana*)

Lower your forehead to the mat and reach your hands back to hold on to your heels. Keep your forehead on the ground as you lift your hips up as high as they will go to stretch along your spine. Hold for ten breaths.

10. Happy Baby Pose (*Ananda Balasana*)

Flip over to lie on your back. Draw your knees in toward your shoulders and press your tailbone into the floor. Stay here or progress into the full version of the pose by stacking your ankles over your knees and holding on to your big toes or the outer edges of your feet. Hold for ten breaths.

11. Corpse Pose (*Savasana*)

Release your knees or feet and extend your arms and legs out on your mat. Soften your shoulders away from your ears, close your eyes, and breathe deeply. Stay here for five minutes or longer.

YOGA SEQUENCE 2
Full Body Vitality

LEVEL: Intermediate   PROPS REQUIRED: Block (optional)

Blossom into spring with this full-body practice for renewal and action. As nature awakens, this is the perfect time for us to shake off the slumber and lethargy of winter with renewed vigor and optimism! This sequence will give you an equal opportunity to work on your strength, flexibility, and balance. Do this flow whenever you want to tap into your own source of vitality and energy.

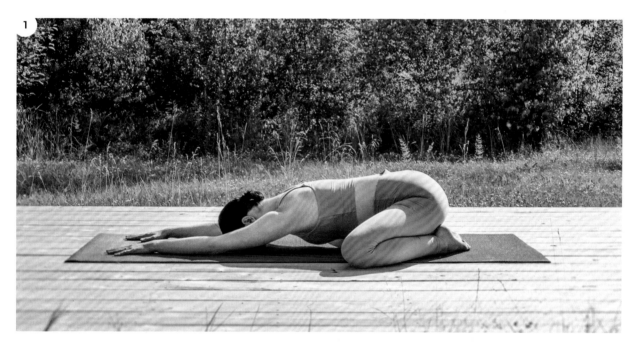

1. Extended Child's Pose (*Utthita Balasana*)
From your hands and knees, widen your knees to the edges of your mat and bring your big toes together to touch. Press your hips back toward your heels and extend your arms forward, gently lowering your forehead to the ground or to a block. Hold for ten breaths.

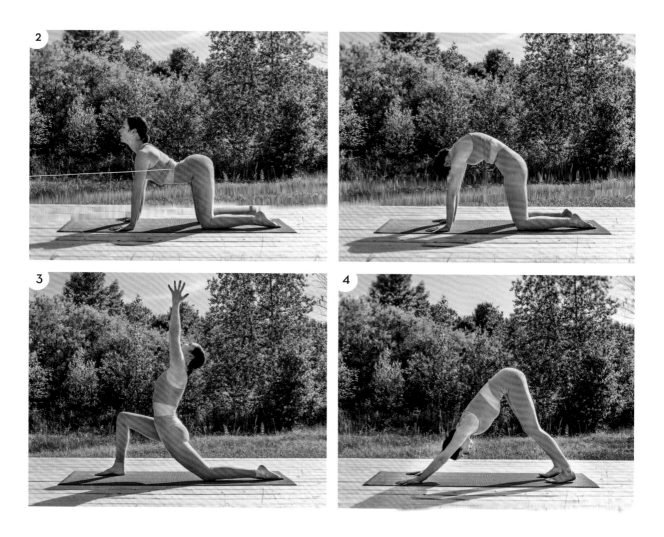

2. Cat/Cow Pose (*Marjaryasana/Bitilasana*)

Come to a table top position. Inhale to arch your back and look up as you stretch the front of your torso. Exhale to reverse this motion by rounding your back and dropping your head to stretch along your spine. Move in and out of these two poses for ten breath cycles.

3. Low Lunge Pose (*Anjaneyasana*)

Step your right foot forward between your palms, aligning your knee over your ankle. Raise your arms up overhead and press your palms together, gazing at your thumbs. Hold for five breaths before switching sides.

4. Downward-Facing Dog Pose
(*Adho Mukha Svanasana*)

From all fours, walk your hands a few inches past your shoulders. Tuck your toes under and lift your hips up and back. Reach your chest toward your thighs and relax your neck. Hold for ten breaths.

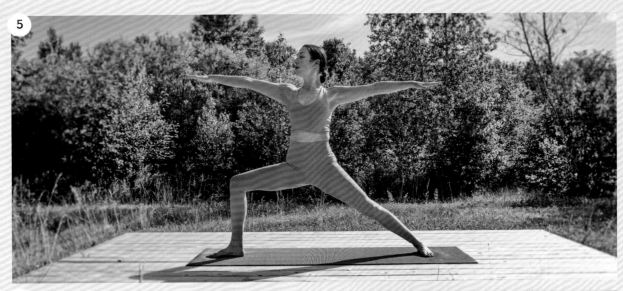

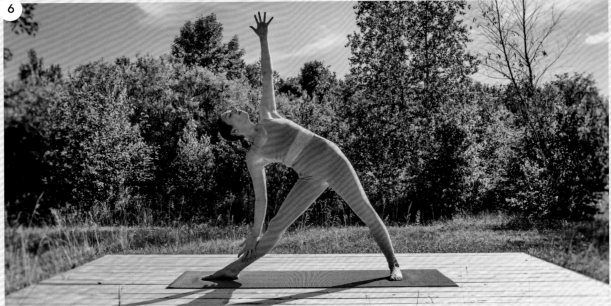

5. Warrior 2 Pose (*Virabhadrasana II*)

Step your right foot to the top of your mat and align your left foot parallel to the back of your mat. Bend your right knee generously and extend your right arm forward and left arm backward with your palms facing down. Gaze over your right hand and hold for five breaths.

6. Triangle Pose (*Trikonasana*)

Straighten your right leg and shorten your stance by bringing your back foot in a few inches. Reach your right arm forward and down to press the back of your hand on your inner right shin. Extend your left arm up and hold for ten breaths.

7. Standing Pigeon Pose (*Tada Kapotasana*)

Step to the top of the mat. Lift your chest up and balance on your right leg. Cross your left ankle over the top of your right thigh. Bring your hands to your heart and bend your right knee as you shift your hips back. Hold for ten breaths.

8. Vinyasa (see pages 20–21)

Release the Standing Pigeon pose and flow through a vinyasa.

Repeat Warrior 2, Triangle, and Standing Pigeon poses on the second side. Follow with a vinyasa.

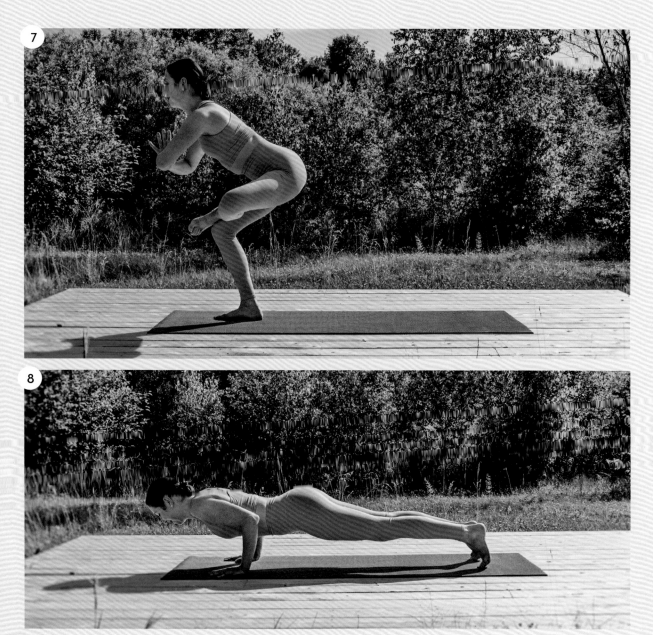

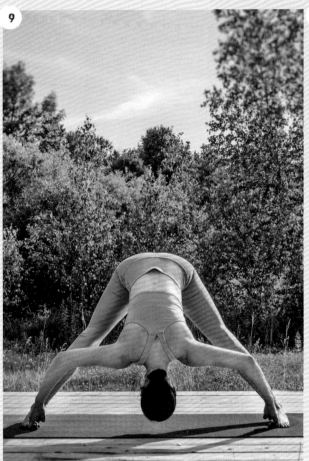

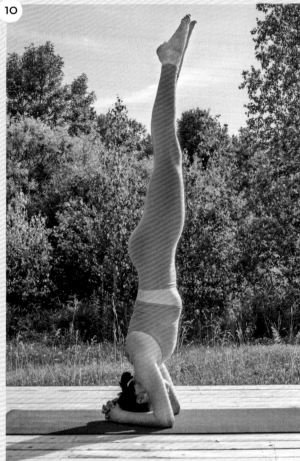

9. Wide-Legged Forward Bend Pose
(*Prasarita Padottanasana*)

Stand up and open your legs wide, aligning your feet so they are parallel to the shorter edges of your mat. Bring your hands to your hips and hinge forward to fold down, reaching the crown of your head toward the mat. Choose to place your hands on the mat or reach for your big toes. Hold for ten breaths.

10. Supported Headstand Pose (*Salamba Sirsasana*)

Interlace your fingers and place your forearms on the ground. Gently place the crown of your head between your elbows. Align your hips over your shoulders and stay here or lift your legs up toward the sky for the full expression of the pose. Engage your core and push your arms into the ground to take the weight off your neck. Hold for ten breaths.

11. Bridge Pose (*Setu Bandha Sarvangasana*)

Lower all the way down onto your back. Bend your knees and place your feet flat on the floor close to your seat. Roll your shoulders away from your ears and extend your arms by your sides with your palms facing up on the mat. Push your feet into the ground to lift your hips up high. Hold for ten breaths.

12. Reclined Butterfly Pose (*Supta Baddha Konasana*)

Bring the soles of your feet together to touch and let your knees fall open. Close your eyes and take ten deep breaths in and out through your nose.

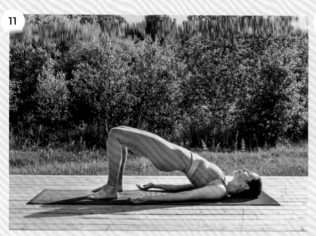

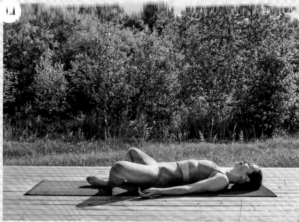

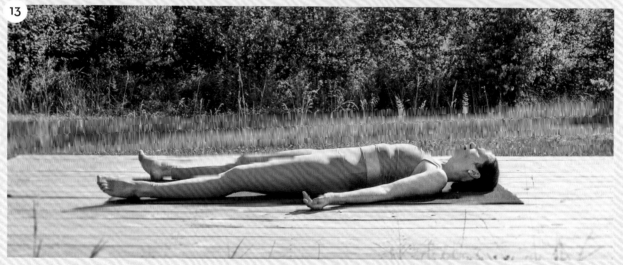

13. Corpse Pose (*Savasana*)

Stretch your arms and legs out on your mat. Relax your shoulders away from your ears, close your eyes, and breathe deeply. Stay here for five minutes or longer.

YOGA SEQUENCE 3
Yin Yoga for Confidence

LEVEL: Intermediate   **PROPS REQUIRED:** 2 blocks or a bolster (optional)

Yin yoga incorporates the teachings of traditional Chinese medicine with yoga poses that stimulate the flow of qi through the meridian lines.

This sequence is meant to help you trust yourself and connect to your inner power with poses that target the kidney and bladder meridians. An unbalanced kidney meridian line can lead to fear and insecurity. An unbalanced bladder meridian line can lead to indecisiveness.

When both are in balance, they provide us with energy, self-assurance, self-esteem, and confidence. This sequence will target your inner thighs, spine, and hamstrings, where these meridian lines travel. Remember not to go too far into each stretch and relax your muscles as much as possible.

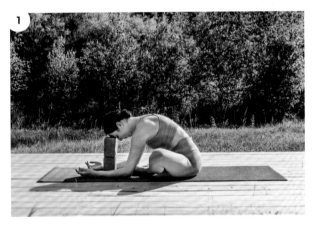

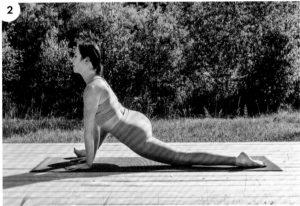

1. Butterfly Pose

Sit up and bring the soles of your feet together to touch. Hinge from your hips to fold forward, allowing your spine to naturally round. You can use two blocks or a bolster under your chest and forehead or simply let gravity pull you deeper into the pose. Hold for three to five minutes.

2. Winged Dragon Pose

Come onto your hands and knees and step your right foot forward to the outer edge of your right palm. Roll onto the edge of your right foot to externally rotate your hip. Stay up on your palms or go deeper by lowering onto your forearms. You can place your blocks or bolster under your head and chest for more support. Hold the pose for three to five minutes before switching sides.

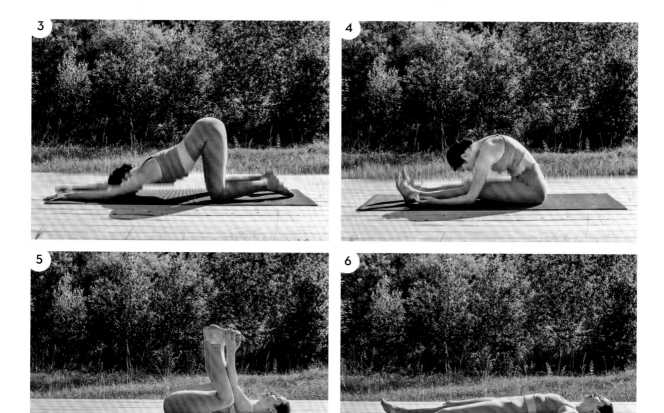

3. Melting Heart Pose

From your hands and knees, walk your hands out in front of you as lower your forehead to the mat or a block. Keep your hips over your knees and melt your heart toward the earth. Hold for three to five minutes.

4. Caterpillar Pose

Come to a sitting position with your legs extended out in front of you. Walk your hands out to fold over your thighs, bending your knees slightly if needed. Let your head be heavy and relax your shoulders away from your ears. Hold for three to five minutes.

5. Happy Baby Pose

Lower onto your back and draw your knees in toward your shoulders. Stay here or progress into the full version of the pose by stacking your ankles over your knees and holding on to your big toes or the edges of your feet. Hold for three to five minutes.

6. Corpse Pose

Extend your legs out one at a time, bringing your feet toward the corners of your mat. Soften your shoulders away from your ears as you relax your arms by your sides with your palms facing up. Close your eyes and breathe deeply, holding the pose for five minutes or longer.

YOGA SEQUENCE 4
Yoga for Neck & Shoulder Pain

LEVEL: Beginner   **PROPS REQUIRED:** Strap (optional)

With the warmer weather, you might find yourself doing outdoor activities like hiking or gardening more often. If that's the case, some tension could build up in your upper body. If you're feeling tightness and discomfort in your neck, shoulders, and upper back, this simple sequence will help you feel more at ease. This is a gentle practice that uses primarily seated poses. You could even do some of these stretches whenever you feel stiff while sitting at a desk.

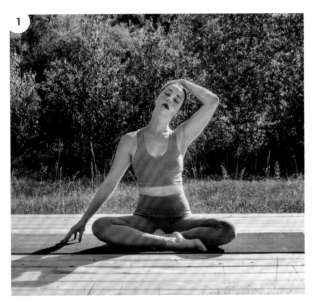

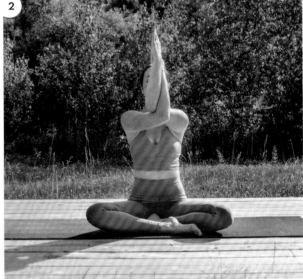

1. Seated Neck Release

Sit cross-legged with your spine lifted tall. Drop your left ear to your left shoulder and slide your shoulder blades down your back. Use your left hand to pull your right ear away from your right shoulder. Take ten breaths here before switching sides.

2. Seated Eagle Pose (*Garudasana*)

Bend your elbows at a 90-degree angle in front of you with your palms facing each other. Wrap your right arm under your left arm and wrap your right wrist over your left to press your hands together. Keep your elbows lifted and tuck your chin to your chest. Hold for ten breaths and repeat on the other side.

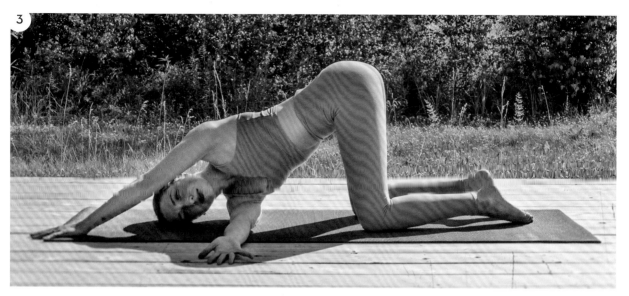

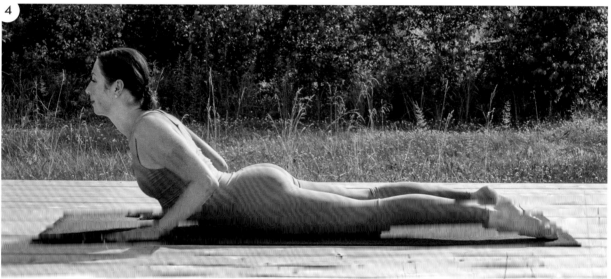

3. Thread the Needle Pose (*Parsva Balasana*)

Come to a Table Top position on all fours. Reach your right arm underneath you toward the left side of your mat with your palm facing up. Lower your right shoulder and ear to the mat. Extend your left arm up overhead. Push your right arm and your left hand into the floor. Hold for ten breaths before switching sides.

4. Cobra Pose (*Bhujangasana*)

Lower to your belly and place your hands next to your rib cage. Push into your palms to lift your chest off the mat. Squeeze your elbows toward your body and roll your shoulders back. Hold for three breaths and repeat two more times.

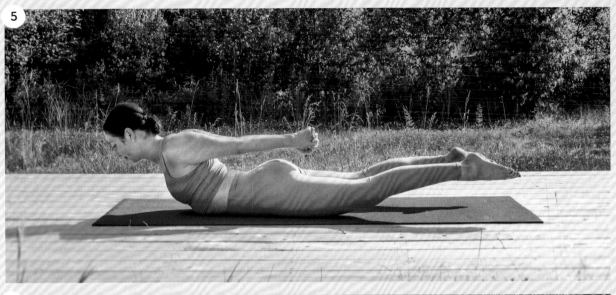

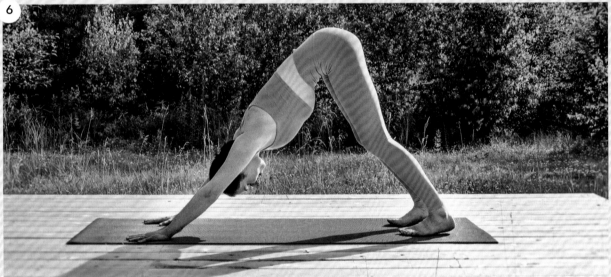

5. Locust Pose (*Salabhasana*)

Interlace your hands behind your lower back. As you inhale, lift your chest and legs off the mat. Tuck your chin in slightly to elongate your neck and press your pelvis into the floor. Lift your hands off your lower back. Hold for five breaths and repeat once more, looping your hands the other way.

6. Downward-Facing Dog Pose
(*Adho Mukha Svanasana*)

Press up into a Table Top pose and walk your hands a few inches past your shoulders. Tuck your toes under and lift your hips up and back. Put the emphasis on sliding your shoulder blades down your back and relaxing your neck completely. Hold for ten breaths.

7. Standing Forward Bend Pose Variation (*Uttanasana*)

Walk your feet to the top of the mat so that your upper body dangles over your legs. Bend your knees as much as is comfortable. Relax your neck and hold on to your upper arms as you sway from side to side. Hold for ten breaths.

8. Cow Face Pose (*Gomukhasana*)

Come down to a seated position. Wrap your right leg over your left in order to stack your right knee over the left one. Place your right palm on your upper back with your elbow pointing up. Reach for your right fingertips with your left hand or use a strap to make it easier. Hold for ten breaths before switching sides.

9. Corpse Pose (*Savasana*)

Lower onto your back and bring your arms beside your body with your palms facing up and your legs out straight. Relax your shoulders away from your ears, close your eyes, and breathe deeply. Stay for five minutes or longer.

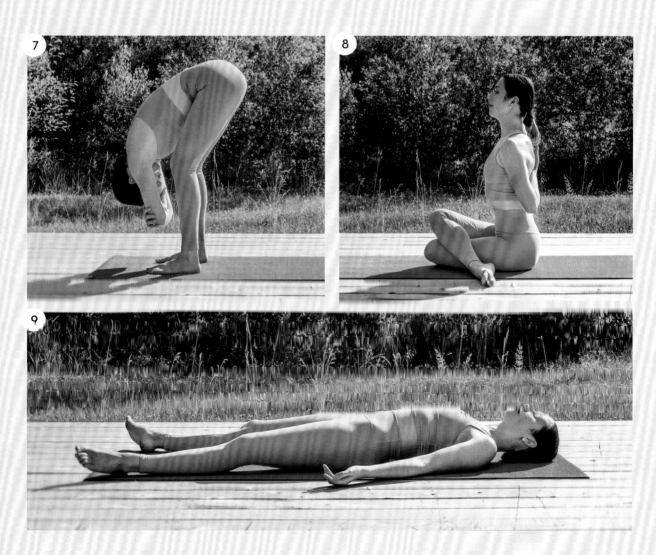

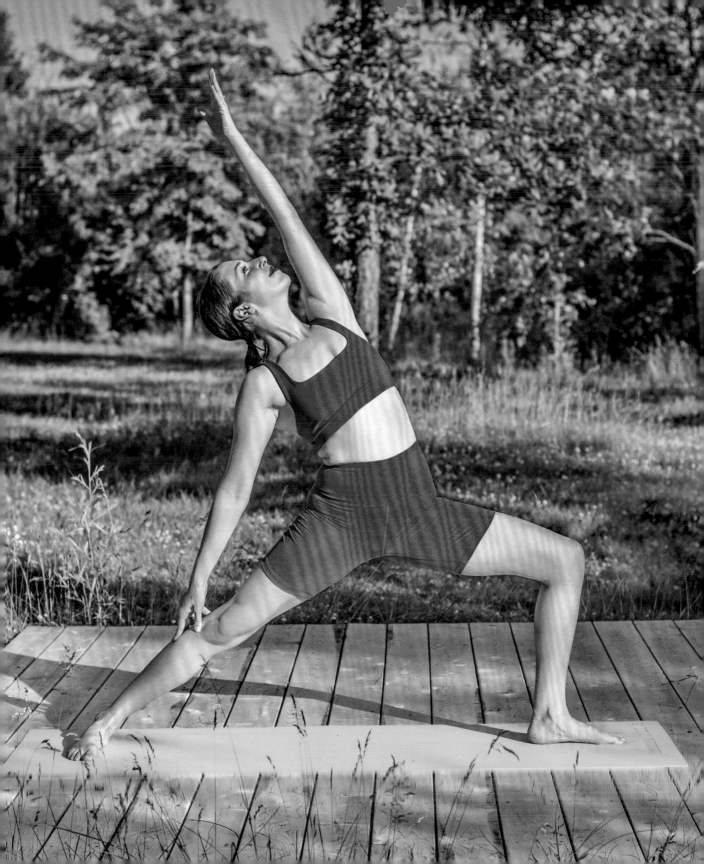

SUMMER

>)))))))) ● ● ● ((((((((

Warm summer sun,
Shine kindly here,
Warm southern wind,
Blow softly here.
Green sod above,
Lie light, lie light.
Good night, dear heart,
Good night, good night.

—Mark Twain

>)))))))) ● ● ● ((((((((

The energy of summer is one of celebration! The flowers are blooming, and all of nature is awake and vibrant. The practices in this section will support you in making the most of this dynamic time.

You've worked hard this year, so be proud of yourself and how far you have come. Celebrate with loved ones and begin and end your day with a grateful heart.

THEME: bloom and celebrate

WORDS: abundance, connection, forgiveness, blooming, peak, fertility, manifesting, generosity, culmination, overflow, caring, compassion, vibrancy, gathering

FEELINGS: gratitude, elation, contentment

BEST TIME TO: Go out and socialize with friends and family. Make love, create art, celebrate, and give freely. Stay up late, possibly for a moon bath. Practice vigorous forms of yoga. Build a fire, get messy, paint, and generally, have fun!

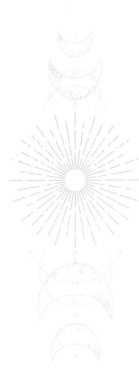

MORNING PRACTICE
Sun Salutations

LEVEL: All Levels   **PROPS REQUIRED:** None

Summer is a celebration of longer days, warmth, and sunshine. What better way to show gratitude for this than by beginning our mornings with a few rounds of *Surya Namaskar* (Sun Salutation)!

Sun salutations gracefully link together a series of asanas (yoga poses) and provide the student with an excellent cardiovascular workout. They also help build full body strength and flexibility—all in all, the perfect short morning flow!

This particular form of sun salutation comes from the Ashtanga Vinyasa lineage. Each pose is held for only one part of the breath. If the weather allows, I encourage you to do this practice outdoors, perhaps even at sunrise.

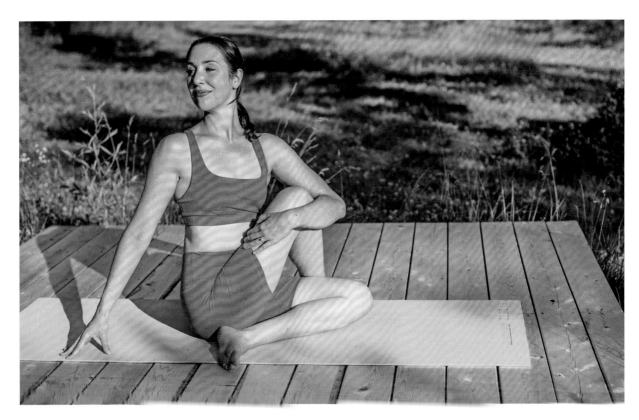

1. Mountain Pose (*Tadasana*)

Stand up tall at the top of your mat with your feet hip-width apart. Roll your shoulders back and turn your palms forward. Push into all four corners of both feet. Exhale fully.

2. Raised Arm Pose (*Urdhva Hastasana*)

Inhale to reach your arms up overhead. Bring your palms together as you look up.

3. Standing Forward Bend Pose (*Uttanasana*)

Exhale to fold forward toward your toes. Bend your knees as much as you need to in order to protect your lower back.

4. Standing Half Forward Bend Pose (*Ardha Uttanasana*)

Inhale to lift your chest up halfway, parallel to the mat. Place your fingertips on the mat in front of you or on your shins if needed. Roll your shoulders back and keep the weight in your toes.

5. Four-Limbed Staff Pose (*Chaturanga Dandasana*)

Exhale to step your feet back into Plank pose and bend your elbows to a 90-degree angle. Keep your upper arms close to your rib cage and your core engaged. You can make this easier by lowering your knees to the mat. Intermediate and advanced students can hop the feet back into Four-Limbed Staff pose immediately and skip the Plank pose.

6. Upward-Facing Dog Pose (*Urdhva Mukha Svanasana*)

Inhale to roll over your toes and lift your chest up you straighten your arms. Squeeze the muscles in your legs to keep your knees and pelvis lifted off the ground. If this is difficult for you, do Cobra pose (*Bhujangasana*) instead with your elbows bent and your hips on the mat.

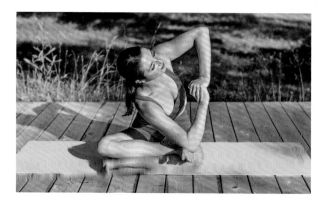

7. Downward-Facing Dog Pose (*Adho Mukha Svanasana*)

Exhale to lift your hips up and back into Downward-Facing Dog. Your feet should be hip-width distance apart with your hands shoulder-width apart. Bend your knees as much as you'd like as you reach your tailbone up.

8. Standing Half Forward Bend Pose (*Ardha Uttanasana*)

From Downward-Facing Dog, bend your knees to look at the top of the mat. Step or hop your feet in between your palms and inhale to find your Standing Half Forward Bend pose once more.

9. Standing Forward Bend Pose (*Uttanasana*)

Exhale to fold forward.

10. Raised Arm Pose (*Urdhva Hastasana*)

Inhale as you come all the way up to standing, leading with your chest and ending your arms up overhead.

11. Mountain Pose (*Tadasana*)

Exhale back into your standing position. Repeat for four to nine more rounds as is appropriate for your body.

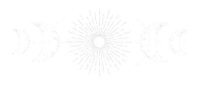

1. and 11. Mountain Pose (*Tadasana*)

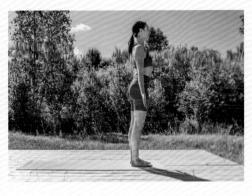

10. Raised Arm Pose (*Urdhva Hastasana*)

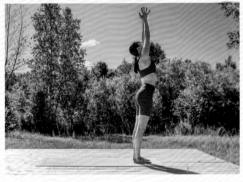

9. Standing Forward Bend Pose (*Uttanasana*)

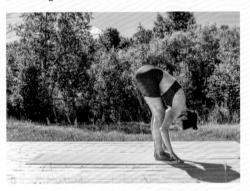

8. Standing Half Forward Bend Pose (*Ardha Uttanasana*)

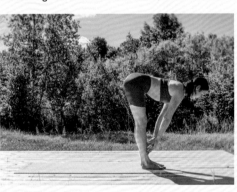

7. Downward-Facing Dog Pose (*Adho Mukha Svanasana*)

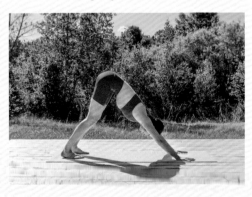

2. Raised Arm Pose (*Urdhva Hastasana***)**

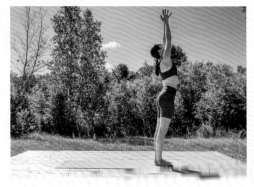

3. Standing Forward Bend Pose (*Uttanasana***)**

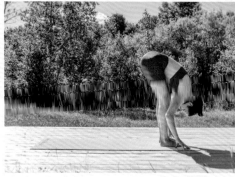

4. Standing Half Forward Bend Pose (*Ardha Uttanasana***)**

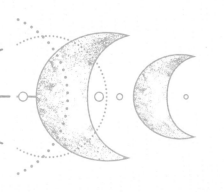

5. Four-Limbed Staff Pose (*Chaturanga Dandasana***)**

6. Upward Facing Dog Pose (*Urdhva Mukha Svanasana***)**

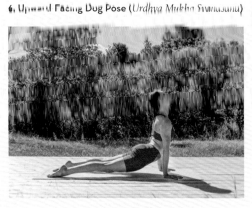

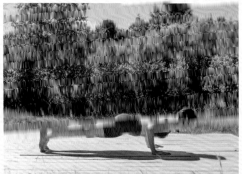

EVENING MEDITATION

Mantra Meditation

One of my favorite meditation techniques involves the use of a mantra—an incantation of words of power—repeated internally as a point of focus. This is a great way to reduce the amount of internal noise that takes us out of a meditative state.

The concept is simple: We simply merge each part of the breath with a part of the mantra. The one we'll be using in our summer evening meditation is *So Hum*, which can be translated to *So*, "That," and *Hum*, "I," or "I Am That."

Vedic teachings explain that So in the mantra represents oneness with the universe and the great force behind all of creation. It is a wonderful sound to employ when we desire to connect to the part of ourselves that is greater than our physical bodies. It also speaks to the interconnected nature of all beings.

You can use *dhyana mudra* during this meditation to facilitate stillness of mind. This mudra, or hand gesture, is known as the mudra of concentration and meditation. Your hands form the shape of a triangle, which represents the three jewels of Buddhism: Buddha (the teacher, the enlightened one), Dharma (the teachings, good law), and Sangha (community).

1. *Sit comfortably with your shoulders relaxed and your eyes closed.*
2. *Use* dhyana mudra *by placing your hands in your lap, right over left with palms facing up and both thumbs touching.*
3. *Relax your breath to a sustainable soft rhythm. Relax your facial muscles.*
4. *As you inhale through your nose, internally repeat So.*
5. *As you exhale out your nose, internally repeat Hum.*

You may wish to use a timer for this meditation. Start with five minutes and work your way up to a longer practice.

If you notice your mind beginning to wander, don't judge or label the experience; simply come back to the mantra and to the breath. Tune in to your own connection with this mantra and the way it connects you to your true essence.

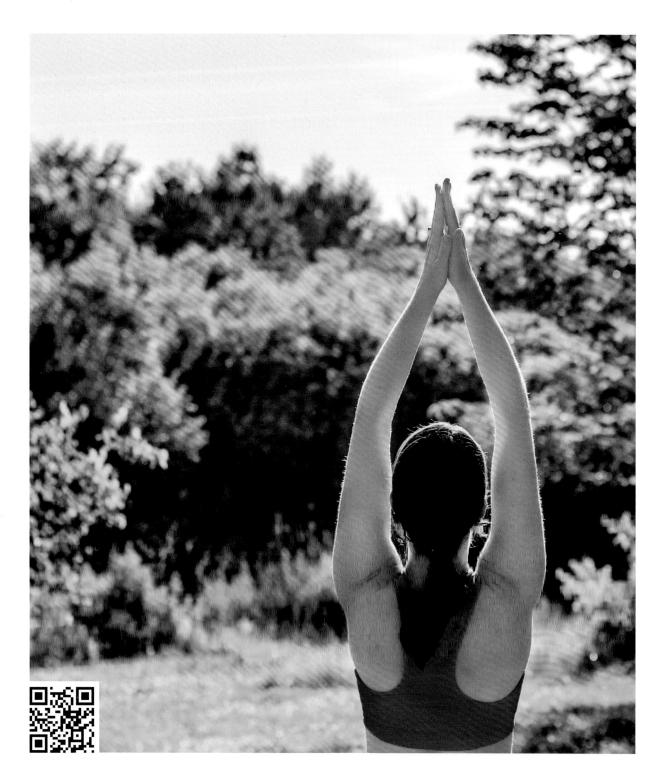

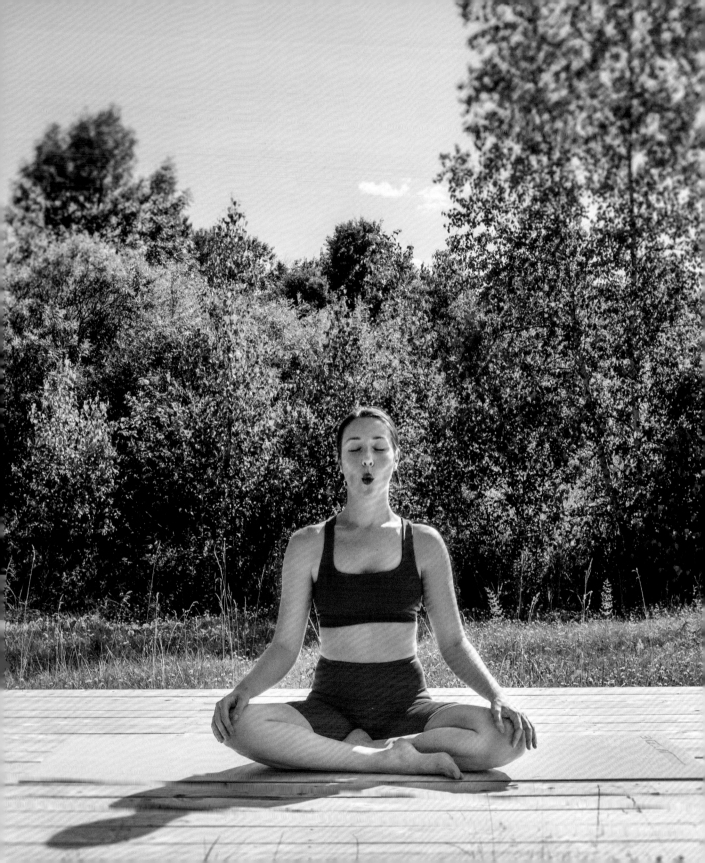

BREATHING EXERCISE

Sitali Pranayama

One of the most powerful tools we have at our disposal is our breath. Some breathing techniques allow us to calm our nervous system, others help us focus and concentrate. The breathing exercise featured here, *sitali pranayama*, helps us cool down.

As the heat increases during the summer, utilize this technique to cool your inner fire. This is a wonderful practice to do after an invigorating or sweaty yoga practice, in the afternoon when the sun is hottest, or anytime you feel your own internal fire burning too hot.

To perform this pranayama, sit in a comfortable position and lengthen your spine. Close your eyes and make an "O" shape with your mouth. Stick your tongue out of your mouth and curl it lengthwise, creating a cylindrical shape.

1. *Inhale deeply through your mouth as if you were drinking from a straw. Notice the cool air on your tongue and imagine it flowing like a breeze all the way down to your belly. This breath should feel easy and comfortable, never forced. You might inhale for a count of four, five, or six.*

2. *Hold your breath at the top of the inhale for a count or two*

3. *Bring your tongue back in and close your mouth to exhale through your nose. Exhale for that same count of four, five, or six.*

4. *Hold the breath out at the end of the exhale for a count or two*

5. *Repeat the first four steps for two to five minutes*

When you're done, relax your jaw and facial muscles and breathe at a rhythm that is comfortable to you. Take a few minutes here before resuming your day.

AFFIRMATIONS

Rejoice in the summer season with these positive affirmations for joy, abundance, and connection. Whether you choose to repeat the affirmations internally or out loud, notice the thoughts and feelings that arise within you.

Some affirmations might feel effortless and natural; others might bring up resistance and doubt. It's important to refrain from any judgment or unkind feelings toward yourself. All of this is valuable feedback for your reflection. Journaling can help you understand your feelings further.

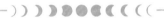

1. *I am blessed, grateful, and abundant.*

2. *I step into my power with confidence and grace.*

3. *I am an open channel for creativity.*

4. *I allow myself to play and be silly.*

5. *I am a vessel of love.*

6. *I am healthy, happy, and radiant.*

7. *Joy is my birthright.*

8. *In this moment, all is well.*

9. *There is plenty for everyone, including me.*

10. *I'm worthy of respect and acceptance.*

11. *Abundance flows freely to me.*

12. *Wellness is my natural state.*

13. *The more love I give, the more I receive.*

14. *I am deeply connected to my heart.*

15. *I see through the eyes of compassion.*

16. *I am creatively fulfilled.*

17. *I'm so proud of how far I've come.*

18. *I fully embrace the whole of myself.*

19. *My inner light shines brightly.*

20. *I find perfect balance between speaking and listening.*

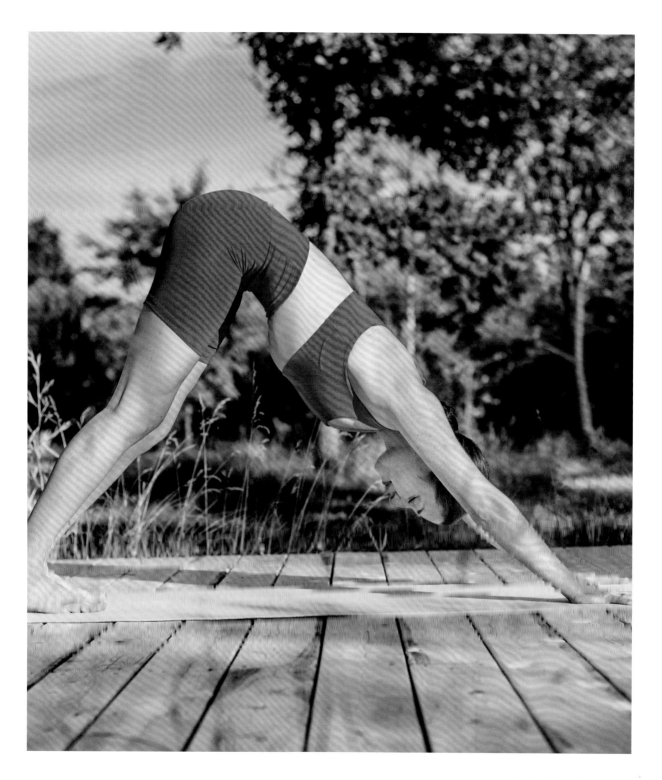

NEW MOON RITUAL

Tea Ritual

A tea ritual is a simple and potent way to tap into the elements of nature and set your intention for the upcoming lunar cycle. As you prepare your brew, you can lovingly infuse it with your intentions and feel the blessing energy as you sip.

Acknowledge and thank each element as you prepare it. The earth element is embodied in the tea leaves themselves. The water element is represented by the water used for the infusion. The fire element comes from boiling your water, and the air element is signified by the steam and aromatic vapors released.

Before you take your first sip, close your eyes and focus on your intention. Repeat it silently or say it out loud to set it.

The great thing about this simple practice is that you can repeat your intention daily throughout the month to remind yourself of what you are calling in. It's an easy way to add some magic to your day.

FULL MOON RITUAL

Moonbathing

Make the most of warm summer nights by spending some time under the light of the full moon. You've probably heard of sunbathing, but moonbathing is just as lovely and much better for your skin.

Summer is associated with fire and the *pitta dosha* in *Ayurveda*, which regulates heat, digestion, energy, and metabolism. Moonbathing is a way of balancing this heat by exposing ourselves to the cooling energy of the moon.

To moonbathe, simply grab a blanket or a yoga mat and lay it out in nature. Lie back in Corpse pose (*Savasana*) or sit in a meditative position and let yourself soak in those healing lunar rays.

To add to the experience, surround yourself with some of the crystals in the summer listicle (page 114) and listen to the Full Moon playlist (page 25). Breathe deeply and listen to the sounds of nature all around you. Stay out as long as you like.

LISTICLE

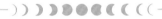

Celebrate the season with these recommended resources for summer. Enjoy this curated playlist for your practices as well as the recommended readings, fresh smoothie recipe, and more.

Music

"Faith's Hymn" by Beautiful Chorus
"Awake" by Tycho
"Follow the Sun" by Xavier Rudd
"Surya Namaskar (Sun Salutation)" by
    Michael Mandrell and Benjy Wertheimer
"Every Morning" by Sugar Ray
"Put Your Records On" by Corinne Bailey Rae
"Lucky" by Jason Mraz and Colbie Caillat
"Nectar Drop" by DJ Drez
"Airwaves" by Ray LaMontagne
"Blue Moon" by Beck
"Gayatri" by Lisbeth Scott

Books

The Mastery of Love by Don Miguel Ruiz
The Bhagavad Gita by the sage Vyasa
The Heart of Yoga by T. K. V. Desikachar
You Can Heal Your Life by Louise Hay
Year of Yes by Shonda Rhimes
Man's Search for Meaning by Viktor Frankl

Crystals

CITRINE: This is the crystal of abundance! Citrine is also associated with confidence and the solar plexus (*Manipura*) chakra. Its orange color is reminiscent of the sun.

AQUAMARINE: Balance the heat of summer with this cool and calm stone that represents steady waters. Think of it as your "go with the flow" ally.

SUNSTONE: Associated with vitality and joy, this crystal is thought to bring goodwill and optimism.

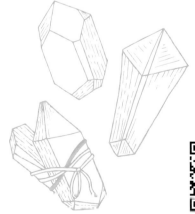

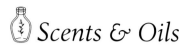 ## Scents & Oils

CINNAMON: This is an invigorating scent that captures the fiery spirit of the season.

LAVENDER: Use this soothing scent when you need to calm down and relax.

CITRONELLA: This refreshing and uplifting scent has the added benefit of being an insect repellent.

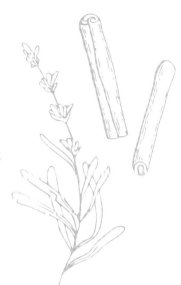

CHAKRA: Solar Plexus *(Manipura)*

ELEMENT: Fire

MOON PHASE: Full Moon

CARDINAL DIRECTION: South

ZODIAC: Cancer, Leo, Virgo

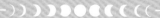

REFRESHING PINEAPPLE & CILANTRO SMOOTHIE RECIPE

SERVES 1 TO 2

1 cup diced pineapple

1 banana

1 cup fresh kale

1 celery stalk

Handful freshly chopped cilantro

1 cup water

¼ cup ice (optional)

Combine all ingredients in a blender and add ice if desired. Blend until desired consistency is reached. Replace the water with 1 cup of nondairy milk to thicken the smoothie and make it creamier. You also can replace the cilantro with basil if desired.

YOGA SEQUENCE 1
Fire Element

LEVEL: Intermediate   **PROPS REQUIRED:** Block

Summer is all about heat and the power of fire. Fire is associated with the solar plexus (*Manipura*) chakra, located in the abdomen. This strong sequence is a wonderful way to honor the element of fire associated with transformation, determination, passion, and energy.

This practice is designed to stoke the fire within and build internal heat through core strength, twists, and side bends. As you flow, focus on your own determination and willpower, even as the poses get challenging.

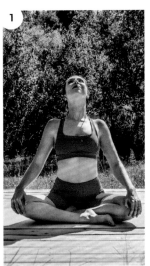
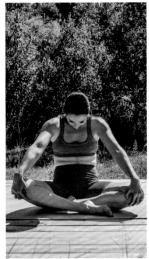

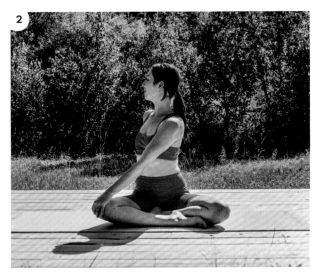

1. Seated Cat/Cow Pose
(*Upavistha Marjaryasana/Bitilasana*)
Sit up tall in a cross-legged position with your hands resting on your knees. Inhale to arch your back and squeeze your shoulder blades together.

Exhale to reverse this motion by rounding your back and dropping your head to stretch along your spine.

Move in and out of these two poses for ten breath cycles.

2. Easy Twist Pose (*Parivrtta Sukhasana*)
Place your left hand on your right knee and your right hand behind you for support. Lengthen your spine as you inhale and twist over to the right. Exhale as you gaze over your right shoulder. Hold for five breaths before switching sides.

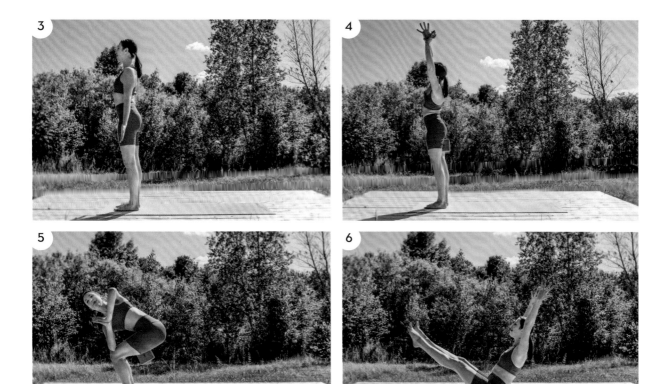

3. Sun Salutations (*Surya Namaskar*)
(see pages 102–105)

Come to a standing position at the top of the mat. Perform five rounds of Surya Namaskar (Sun Salutation).

5. Revolved Chair Pose (*Parivrtta Utkatasana*)

Keep squeezing your block between your thighs and bend your knees as if sitting back in a chair. Place your palms together in prayer and initiate a twist from your torso by placing your right elbow over your left thigh. Hold for ten breaths before switching sides.

4. Standing Side Bend Pose
(*Parsva Urdhva Hastasana*)

Stand at the top of the mat and place your block between your upper inner thighs. Reach your arms up overhead and squeeze your block to engage your adductors. Grab ahold of your right wrist with your left hand and initiate a side bend to the left. Hold for five breaths before switching sides.

6. Boat Pose (*Navasana*)

Continue to squeeze your block between your thighs. From Revolved Chair pose, lower your squat all the way down to the mat until your sit bones make contact with the ground. Lift your legs up and reach your arms up overhead. Straighten your legs for an extra challenge and focus on lifting your chest. Hold for ten breaths.

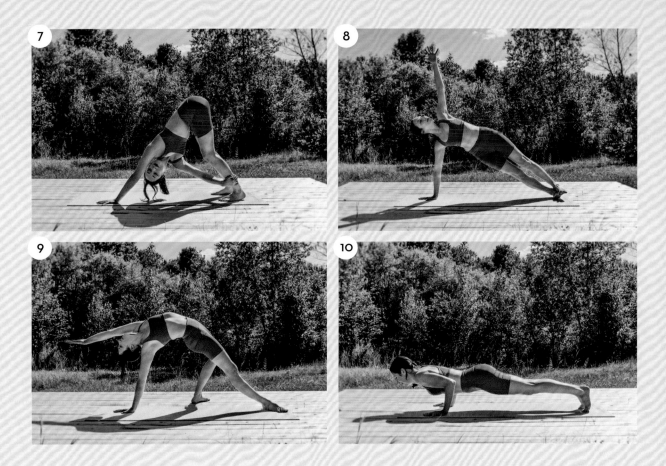

7. Revolved Downward-Facing Dog Pose
(*Parivrtta Adho Mukha Svanasana*)

Release your block and make your way into Downward-Facing Dog pose. Bend your knees in order to bring your right palm to your outer left shin and look under your left shoulder to twist. Straighten your legs any amount and hold for ten breaths before switching sides.

8. Side Plank Pose (*Vasisthasana*)

Shift forward into a Plank pose with your shoulders over your palms. Roll onto the outer edge of your right foot and reach your left arm up to the sky. Hold for five breaths.

9. Wild Thing Pose (*Camatkarasana*)

From your Side Plank pose, step your left foot back behind you and push into both feet to lift your hips up higher. Arch your back and reach your left arm overhead. Hold for five breaths.

10. Vinyasa (see pages 20–21)

Come back through to Plank pose and flow through a vinyasa. Repeat Side Plank and Wild Thing poses on the second side. Follow with a vinyasa.

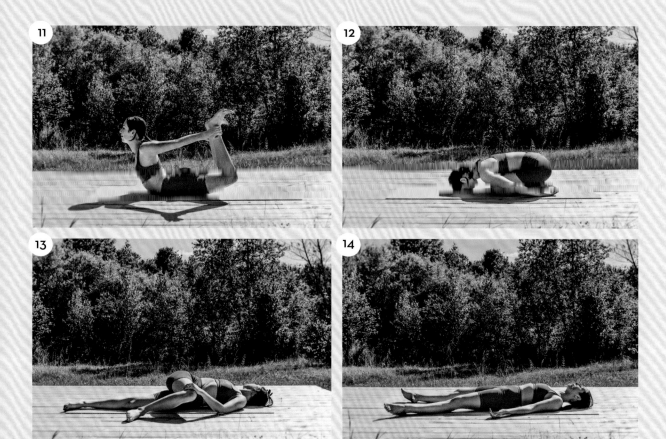

11. Bow Pose (*Dhanurasana*)

Lower to your belly. Bend your knees and reach your arms back to hold on to your outer ankles. Lift your chest and thighs off the mat while squeezing your shoulder blades in. Hold your chest for ten breaths.

13. Reclined Spinal Twist Pose
(*Supta Matsyendrasana*)

Lower all the way down to your back. Pull your right knee into your chest and extend your left leg straight. Cross your right thigh over your chest with the help of your left hand and extend your right arm out to the side. Gaze over your right shoulder and hold for ten breaths before switching sides.

12. Child's Pose (*Balasana*)

Release Bow pose and shift your hips back toward your heels with your knees hip-width apart. Reach your arms back behind you and rest your forehead on the mat. Hold for ten breaths.

14. Corpse Pose (*Savasana*)

Release the twist and stretch your legs and arms out, turning your palms toward the sky. Relax your shoulders away from your ears, close your eyes, and breathe deeply. Stay for five minutes or longer.

YOGA SEQUENCE 2
Yoga for Endurance

LEVEL: Intermediate to Advanced	PROPS REQUIRED: None

Can you keep your cool while under pressure? This sequence is one of my favorite ways to embody and practice the *niyama* of *tapas*. The *yama* and *niyama* come from Patanjali's Yoga Sutras and provide us with a code of ethics and morals. Simply put, the *yama* are things not to do or restraints, while *niyama* are things to do or observances.

The word *tapas* means heat or fire and is commonly understood as austerity, self-discipline, and determination. According to Patanjali, putting the body through intense heat is a way of purifying it. This sequence is designed to generate lots of heat, which can challenge you both mentally and physically. Do your best to stay balanced and centered as you work on this niyama.

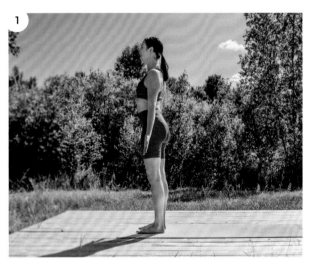

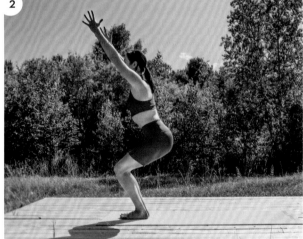

1. Sun Salutations (*Surya Namaskar*)
(see pages 102–105)
Begin with ten rounds of Sun Salutations.

2. Chair Pose (*Utkatasana*)
Bring your big toes together to touch and bend your knees deeply, as if sitting in a chair. Keep your weight in your heels and keep your chest lifted. Reach your arms up overhead. Hold for ten breaths.

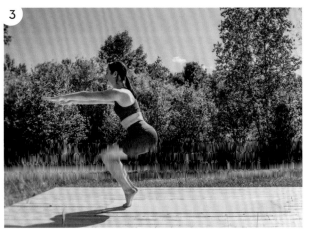

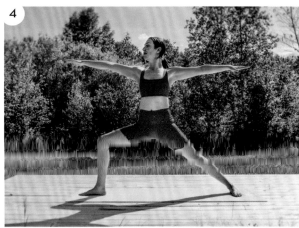

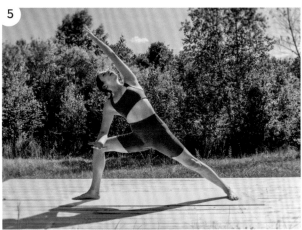

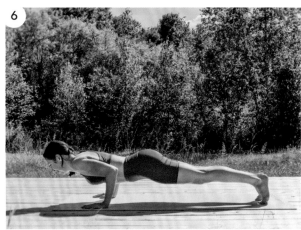

3. Chair Pose Variation (*Utkatasana*)

Bring your arms parallel to the ground and shift your weight onto the balls of your feet. Slowly lift your heels off the mat and hug your inner ankles and thighs together to balance. Sit down even lower and hold for ten breaths.

5. Extended Side Angle Pose
(*Utthita Parsvakonasana*)

Lower your right forearm to your right thigh or to the ground for an extra challenge. Reach your left arm up overhead, making a diagonal line from your left fingertips to your left foot. Hold for ten breaths.

4. Warrior 2 Pose (*Virabhadrasana II*)

Step your left foot back with your foot parallel to the short edge of your mat. Bend your right knee generously and extend your arms out, palms facing down. Gaze over your right hand and hold for ten breaths.

6. Vinyasa (see pages 80–81)

Lower down to Plank pose and flow through a vinyasa.

Repeat Warrior 2 and Extended Side Angle poses on the second side. Follow with a vinyasa.

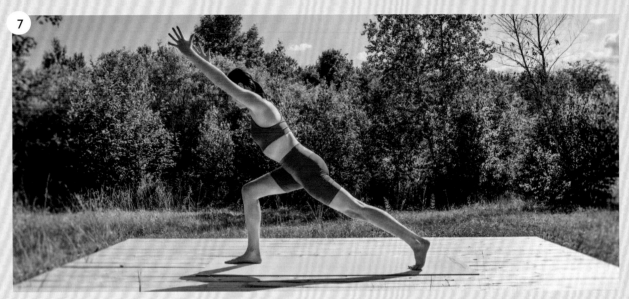

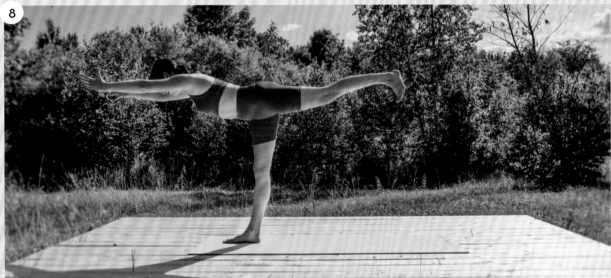

7. High Lunge Pose Variation
(*Ashta Chandrasana*)
Step your right foot forward between your palms and bring your chest and arms up. Bend your front knee to bring your thigh parallel to the mat. Tilt your chest and arms forward, making a diagonal line from your fingertips to your left foot. Hold for ten breaths.

8. Warrior 3 Pose (*Virabhadrasana III*)
Push off of your left foot to balance on your right leg in Warrior 3 pose. Keep your biceps in line with your ears or bring your hands to your heart to make the pose easier. Flex your left foot and roll your left hip down. Hold for ten breaths.

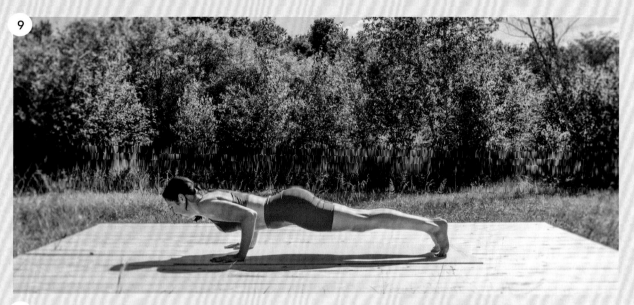

9

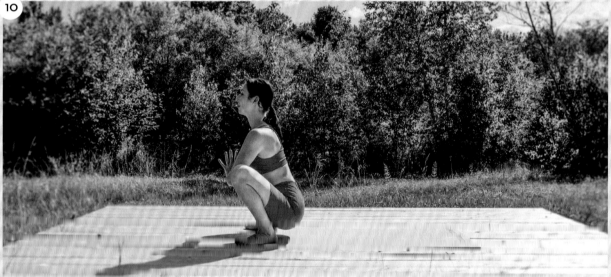

10

9. Vinyasa (see poses 10–01)

Step your left foot back into a lunge. Lower down to Plank
pose and flow through a vinyasa.

Repeat High Lunge Variation and Warrior 3 pose on
the second side. Follow with a vinyasa.

10. Garland Pose (Malasana)

Step your feet hip-width apart with your toes pointed out
at a 45-degree angle. Sit all the way down into a squat position. Bring your hands in prayer at your heart and use your
elbows to press your knees wider. Lengthen your spine and
hold for ten breaths.

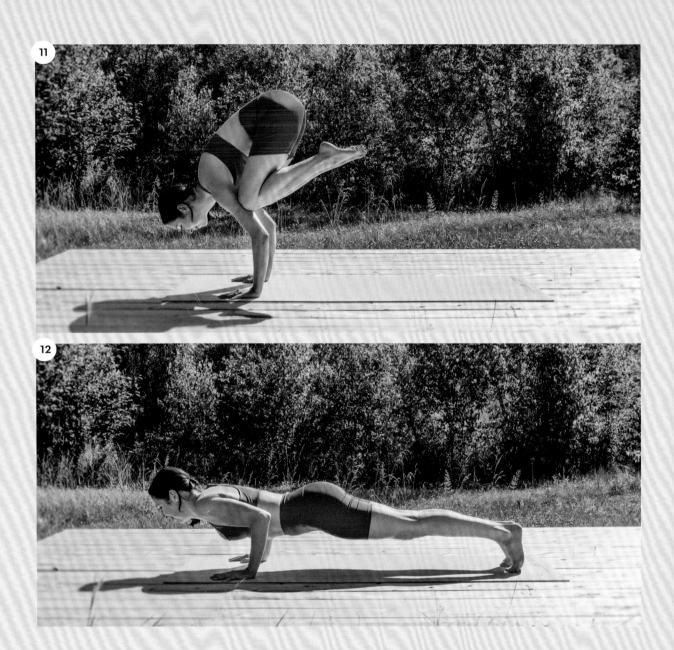

11. Crow Pose (*Bakasana*)

From your squat, place your hands in front of you shoulder-width apart. Lift your hips and place your knees behind your upper arms. Shift your weight into your palms and lift one or both feet off the ground, hugging your inner thighs. Hold for ten breaths.

12. Vinyasa (see pages 20–21)

Step or hop your legs back into Four-Limbed Staff pose to flow through a vinyasa.

13. Reclined Pigeon Pose (*Supta Kapotasana*)

Lower down to your back with your knees bent and feet flat on the floor. Cross your left ankle over your right knee. Reach through with your arms to pull your right thigh toward your chest. Hold for ten breaths and repeat on the other side.

14. Corpse Pose (*Savasana*)

Ease into your final relaxation pose by stretching out your legs and arms and turning your palms toward the sky. Close your eyes and let yourself rest for at least five minutes.

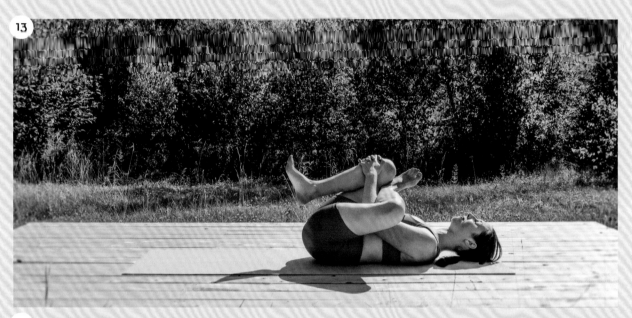

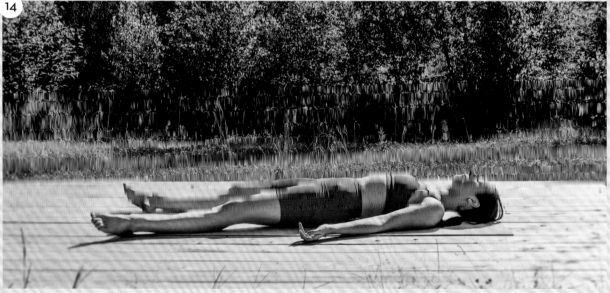

YOGA SEQUENCE 3
Yin Yoga for Joy

LEVEL: Intermediate   **PROPS REQUIRED:** Block and strap (optional)

Yin yoga works with meridian lines by freeing up the flow of qi (energy). This sequence allows you to cultivate more joy by working with the lung and large intestine meridian lines. An unbalanced lung meridian is associated with grief and sadness. An unbalanced large intestine meridian is associated with worry and difficulty letting go.

When both are in balance, we can more easily access feelings of joy, ease, and inner peace. These poses have a strong emphasis on the upper body, as that is where these meridian lines travel.

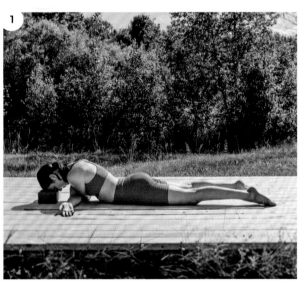

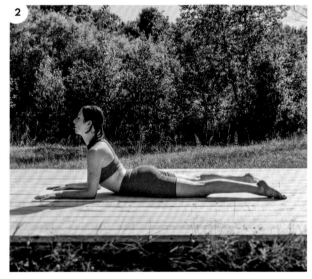

1. Bow Tie Pose

Lie on your stomach and cross your right arm over your left, with both palms facing up. Slide your arms away from one another as far as is comfortable and hold them there. Relax your forehead to the ground or to a block. Hold for three to five minutes.

2. Sphinx Pose

Lift your chest and place your forearms flat on the mat, aligning your elbows under your shoulders. Press your shoulders back and reach your heart forward. Hold for three to five minutes.

Repeat Bow Tie pose, this time crossing your left arm over your right.

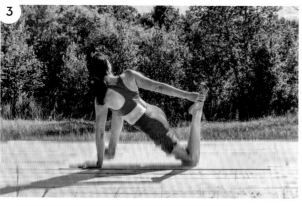

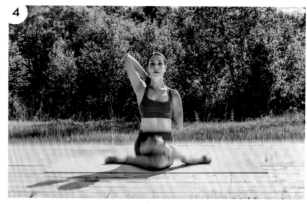

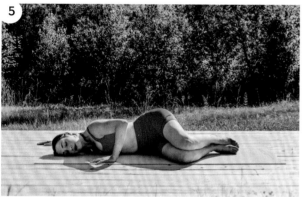

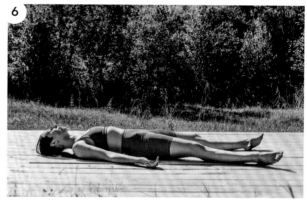

3. Twisted Dragon Pose

Press back onto your hands and knees and step your right foot forward to the top of the mat in a lunge position. Align your right knee over your right ankle and place your left hand on the ground. Reach your right arm back to pull your left ankle toward your glute. Keep your hips low as you pull your heel toward you. Use a strap if needed. Hold for three to five minutes before switching sides.

4. Shoelace with Archer Arms Pose

Take a seat and wrap your right leg over your left in order to stack your right knee over the left one. Place your right palm on your upper back with your elbow pointing up. Reach for your right fingertips with your left hand or use a strap to make it easier. Hold for three to five minutes and repeat on the second side.

5. Broken Wing Pose

Lower to your belly and extend your right arm out to the side with your elbow bent at a 90-degree angle. Align your elbow with your shoulder and roll onto your right side to stretch into your right arm and pectoral muscles. Bend your knees and press your left hand into the floor. Hold for three to five minutes before switching sides.

6. Corpse Pose

Flip over onto your back and extend your limbs out. Soften your shoulders away from your ears as you relax your arms by your sides with your palms facing up. Close your eyes and breathe deeply, holding the pose for five minutes or longer.

YOGA SEQUENCE 4
Yoga for Core Strength

LEVEL: Intermediate   **PROPS REQUIRED:** None

The solar plexus (*Manipura*) chakra, located in our abdomen, is like our own little burning sun. This is the space of our determination, courage, self-esteem, and willpower. Working on core strength is just one of the ways we can stoke this inner fire and tap into those qualities.

Our core includes our abdominal muscles, back, glutes, and hip flexors. This is a strong sequence that can help you improve your posture and balance.

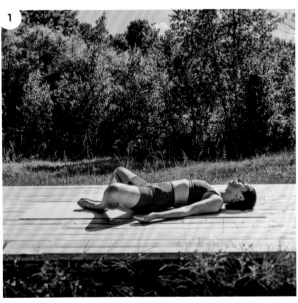

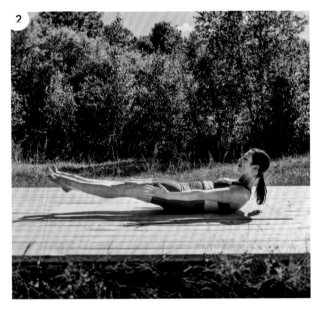

1. Reclined Butterfly Pose (*Supta Baddha Konasana***)**

Lower down onto your back. Bring the soles of your feet together to touch and let your knees fall open. Relax your arms by your sides. Close your eyes and take ten deep breaths in and out through your nose.

2. Low Boat Pose (*Ardha Navasana***)**

Straighten your legs and reach your arms down by your sides. As you inhale, lift your legs, arms, upper back, and head off the mat, making a banana shape with your body. Keep your feet at eye level and draw in your lower belly. Hold for ten breaths. Reach your arms overhead for a greater challenge.

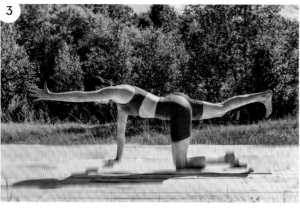

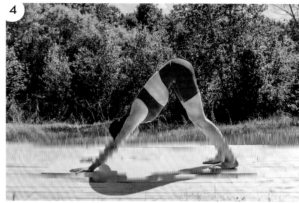

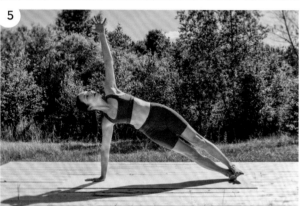

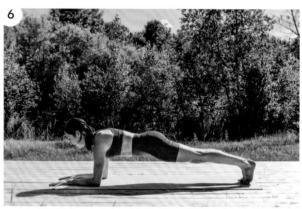

3. Balancing Table Top Pose
(*Dandayamana Bharmanasana*)

Come onto hands and knees in a Table Top pose. Extend your right leg back behind you at hip height. Reach your left arm up with your bicep in line with your ear and gaze down at the mat. Flatten your lower back to engage your abdominal muscles and hold for five breaths before switching sides.

5. Side Plank Pose (*Vasisthasana*)

Shift forward into a Plank pose with your shoulders over your palms. Roll onto the outer edge of your right foot and reach your left arm up to the sky. Hold for five breaths and repeat on the second side.

4. Downward-Facing Dog Pose
(*Adho Mukha Svanasana*)

From Table Top pose, walk your hands a few inches past your shoulders. Tuck your toes under and lift your hips up and back. Reach your chest toward your thighs and press your heels toward the mat. Hold for ten breaths.

6. Dolphin Plank Pose
(*Makara Adho Mukha Svanasana*)

From Plank position, lower down to your forearms, aligning your elbows under your shoulders. Place your palms flat on the floor and keep your hips low, pulling in your lower belly. Hold for ten breaths.

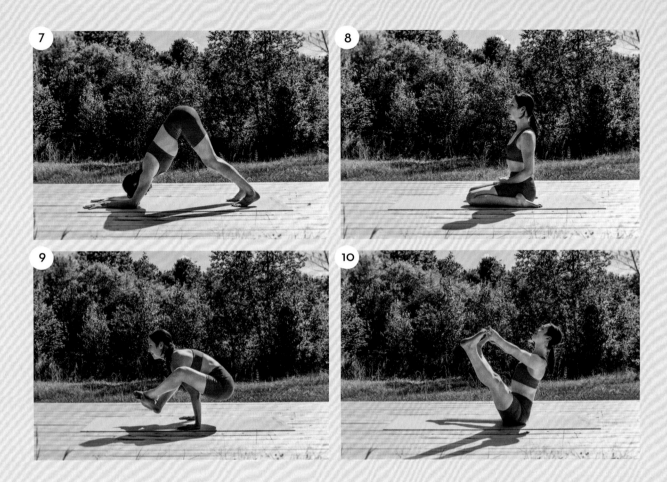

7. Dolphin Pose
(*Ardha Pincha Mayurasana*)

Stay on your forearms and walk your feet in to lift your hips up as high as they will go. Push firmly into the ground with your forearms and press back into your heels. Keep your head lifted off the mat. Hold for ten breaths.

8. Hero Pose (*Virasana*)

Lower your knees to the mat and sit between your shins. Both thigh bones should be parallel to the edges of the mat with your knees hip-width apart. Place your hands on your lap and rest here for ten breaths.

9. Arm Pressure Pose (*Bhujapidasana*)

Bring your legs out in front of you and slide your arms under them. Bring your knees as close to your shoulders as possible. Hook your left ankle over the right and push your palms into the ground to lift your seat. Hold for ten breaths and repeat with the other ankle on top.

10. Upward-Facing Wide-Angle Pose
(*Urdhva Upavistha Konasana*)

Grab your big toes with your peace fingers and rock your weight back onto your sit bones. Lift your chest and extend your legs straight out to the sides. Roll your shoulders back and hold for ten breaths.

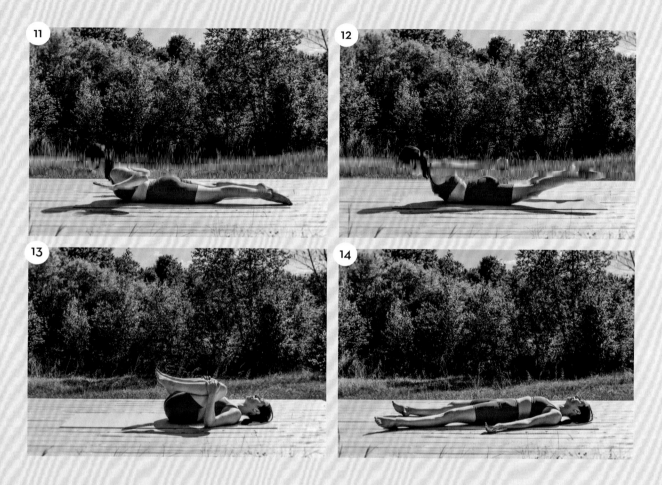

11. Baby Cobra Pose (*Ardha Bhujangasana*)

Lie on your belly and place your palms to the sides of your ribs. Push your pelvis and feet into the floor. As you inhale, lift your palms, chest, and head off the mat, squeezing your elbows in. Exhale to lower back down. Repeat for five breaths.

12. Locust Pose (*Salabhasana*)

Interlace your hands behind your lower back. As you inhale, lift your chest and legs off the mat. Tuck your chin in slightly to elongate your neck and press your pelvis into the floor. Lift your hands off your lower back. Hold for five breaths and repeat once more, clasping your hands the other way.

13. Knees-to-Chest Pose (*Apanasana*)

Flip over onto your back. Draw both knees into your chest, holding on to your shins. Press your tailbone into the ground and gently rock from side to side. Stay for ten breaths.

14. Corpse Pose (*Savasana*)

Release the hold on your knees and stretch your arms and legs out, facing your palms up to the sky. Relax your shoulders away from your ears, close your eyes, and breathe deeply. Stay for five minutes or longer.

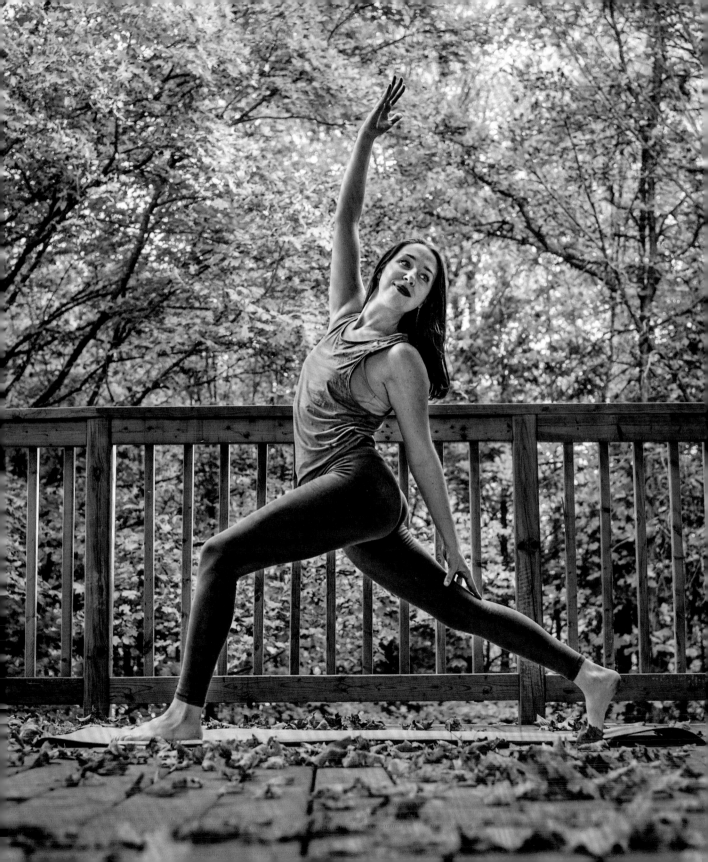

FALL

Autumn whispered to the wind, I fall;
but always rise again.

—Angie Weiland-Crosby

The cycle restarts, and the great wheel of life continues to turn. After the peak of summer comes autumn, a time to wind down and take stock of where we've been, where we are, and where we're going. The trees shed their leaves and so do we. This is an opportunity for us to let go of what no longer serves us.

Continue to work toward the intentions you set at the beginning of the year with renewed precision and purpose. Now is the time to prioritize and focus by dropping the excess and turning inward. Use the practices laid out in this section to support you in this journey.

THEME: release and let go

WORDS: release, boundaries, expelling, clearing out, cleansing, expressing yourself, quitting, forgiving, healing, winding down, harvesting

FEELINGS: introspective, sensitive, inquisitive

BEST TIME TO: Clear the air and clean your house. Set boundaries and let go of what isn't working. Clarify your relationships by expressing yourself. Release trapped emotions through yoga, chanting, journaling, or therapy.

MORNING PRACTICE
Hip Openers

LEVEL: All Levels   **PROPS REQUIRED:** Block and strap (optional)

This season's morning practice is intended to melt away tension from your hips, hamstrings, and lower back. This is a wonderful sequence to do if you spend a lot of time sitting or if you wake up with aches and pains.

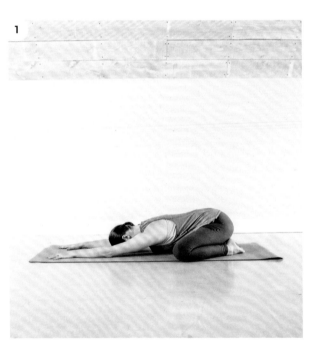

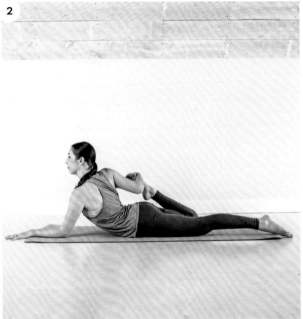

1. Extended Child's Pose (*Utthita Balasana*)
From your hands and knees, widen your knees to the edges of your mat and bring your big toes together to touch. Press your hips back toward your heels and extend your arms forward, gently lowering your forehead to the ground or to a block. Hold for ten breaths.

2. Half Frog Pose (*Ardha Bhekasana*)
Slide onto your belly with your forearms on the mat. Bend your right knee and use your right hand to pull your foot toward your seat. Use a strap if needed. Lift your chest and press your pelvis into the mat. Hold for five breaths before switching sides.

Alleviating physical tension in our bodies is also an excellent way to access and release mental and emotional tension. As you flow through these poses, ask yourself what you want to make space for and what you want to let go of. Set your intention for the day ahead by choosing one word or sentence that captures the essence of how you want to feel, and breathe into it as you go.

3

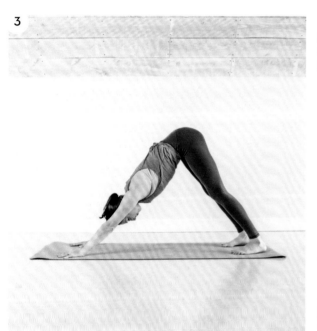

4

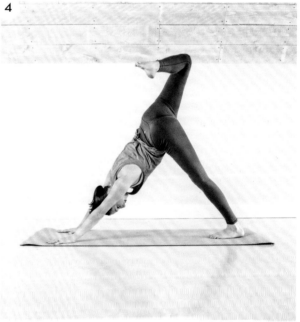

3. Downward-Facing Dog Pose
(*Adho Mukha Svanasana*)

Lift up from your belly onto all fours. Walk your hands a few inches past your shoulders. Tuck your toes under and lift your hips up and back. Reach your chest toward your thighs and relax your neck. Hold for ten breaths.

4. Three-Legged Downward-Facing Dog Pose
Variation (*Eka Pada Adho Mukha Svanasana*)

Lift your right leg up toward the sky and bend your knee to open your hip. Squeeze your right foot toward your seat and hold for five breaths.

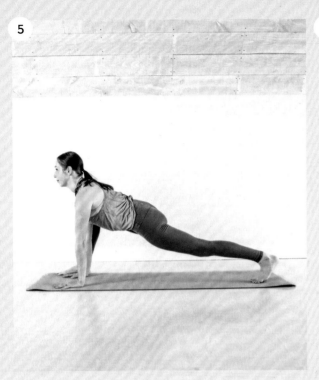

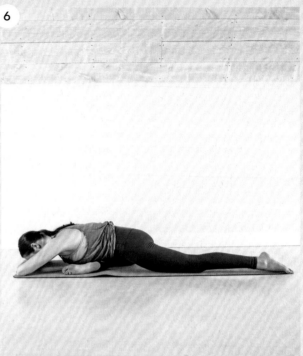

5. Lizard Pose (*Utthan Pristhasana*)

Step your right foot to the outer edge of your right hand. If you can, keep your left knee lifted; if not, lower it to the mat. Intensify the stretch by lowering onto your elbows or stay on your hands for more support. Hold for five breaths.

6. Pigeon Pose (*Ardha Kapotasana*)

From Lizard pose, slide your right foot toward the left side of your mat to place your right knee behind your right wrist. Lower your left knee to the mat and level your hips to avoid tilting to one side. Place a block under your seat for more support. Choose to stay lifted or fold forward over your right shin. Hold for ten breaths.

Step back to Downward-Facing Dog and repeat Three-Legged Downward-Facing Dog, Lizard, and Pigeon poses on the second side.

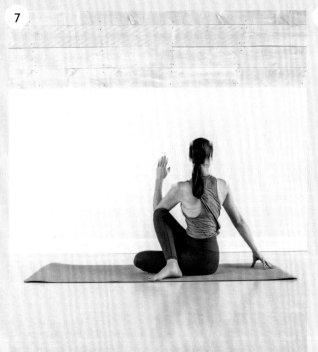

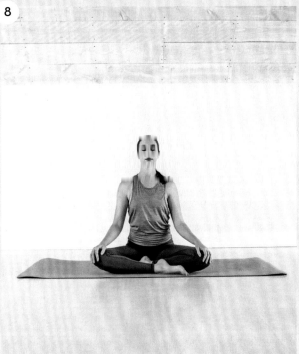

7. Half Lord of the Fishes Pose

(*Ardha Matsyendrasana*)

Come to take a seat with your legs straight out in front of you. Bend your right knee and cross your right foot over your left thigh. Bend your left knee to bring your left foot to your outer right hip. Hook your left elbow to the outside of your right leg and initiate the twist. Hold for five breaths before switching sides.

8. Easy Pose (*Sukhasana*)

Finish this practice by sitting cross-legged on the floor or elevated on a block, resting your hands on your thighs. Close your eyes, focus on the steady rhythm of your breath, and choose your intention for the day. Take ten breaths here.

Bring your palms together at your heart (*anjali mudra*), inhale through your nose, and chant om (*oum*) as you exhale.

EVENING MEDITATION

Body Scan

This season, I'd like to invite you to end your day with a body scan meditation for relaxation. This can be done by sitting on your mat, sitting in a chair, or lying down in bed. The purpose of this guided meditation is to release tension from your body and tune in to the areas that might require a little bit of extra care. Notice sensations as they come and go, and listen to what your body is trying to tell you by noticing the different feelings that arise.

Begin by getting comfortable in either a sitting or lying down position. Close your eyes and breathe deeply in and out through your nose. Focus first on your right foot and move the attention up toward your right thigh, relaxing each muscle along the way. Notice and allow any sensations that might be present in your right leg. Stay here for a few moments before doing the same thing with your left foot and left leg, feeling them get heavier with every breath you take.

If you notice tension in any particular spot, try to breathe into it and imagine the tightness being released as you exhale. Once both feet and legs feel relaxed, focus your attention on your hips and pelvis. Soften into this space. Move your awareness up your back and let your belly be heavy and relaxed as you melt into stillness. Feel the entirety of your torso. Try not to label or judge your experience; simply observe and relax.

Focus next on your right shoulder, relaxing the muscles all the way down your arm and into your right hand. Bring awareness and curiosity to any sensations present there. Repeat the same process with your left shoulder, left arm, and left hand. If your mind begins to wander, bring your focus back to your left arm.

Once both arms are fully relaxed, move up toward your neck and head. Soften your facial muscles and your jaw. Feel the weight of your head and the soft flow of your breath through your nose.

Now, feel the entirety of your body. What is your body trying to communicate to you? Where are sensations coming from and what do they feel like? Is there any part of your body that is still trying to tense and tighten? If so, breathe into it and invite it to let go.

Stay here for as long as you wish, enjoying the total body relaxation. You might drift off to sleep or slowly open your eyes to reawaken and resume your evening.

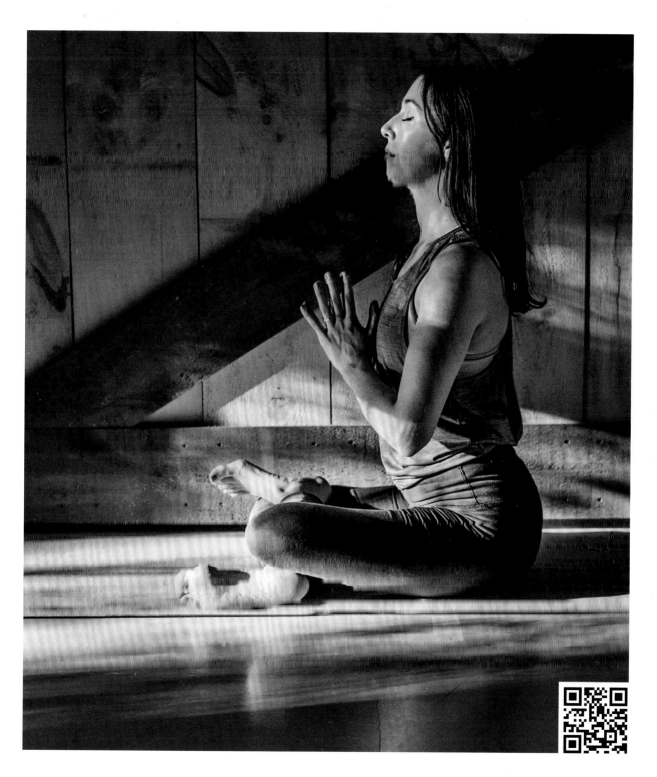

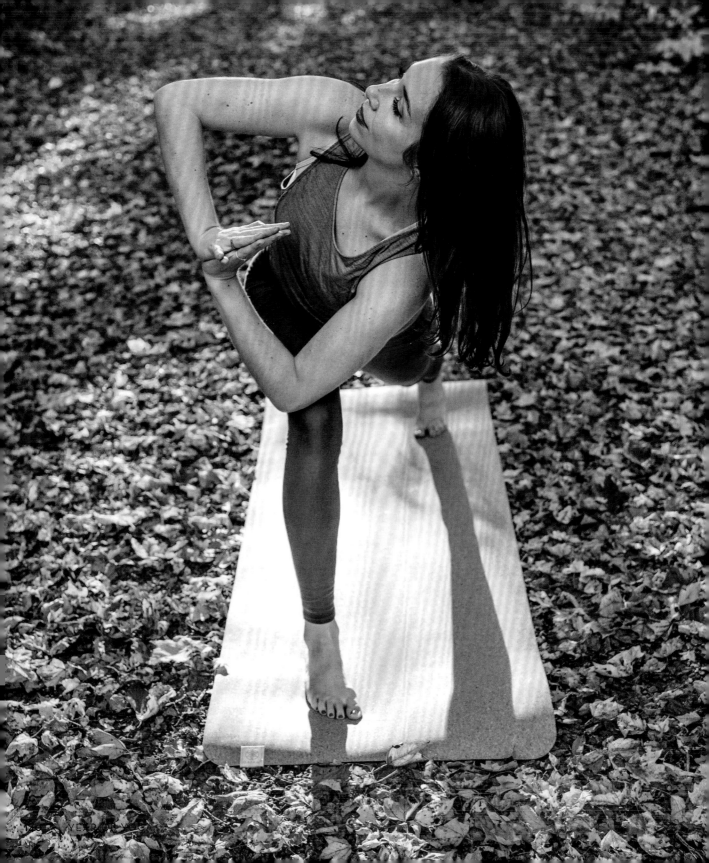

BREATHING EXERCISE

Viloma Pranayama

Whenever I have a hard time falling asleep, this is one of the tools I turn to. *Viloma pranayama* is a breathing technique that facilitates relaxation and helps alleviate stress and anxiety. I recommend doing this one lying down, maybe in your bed before going to sleep at night. It pairs wonderfully with the evening body scan meditation (page 138).

Viloma can be translated as "against the natural order" or "against the wave," and this practice is sometimes called "stair step breathing." There are a few variations of this technique, but my favorite way to practice it is by interrupting the inhales for a few rounds, interrupting the exhales for a few rounds, and finally, interrupting both for a few rounds.

As you practice this, remember that the breath pauses should always feel comfortable and never strained. The pauses should be no more than one to three seconds.

STAGE 1: INTERRUPTED INHALES

Inhale through your nose to fill up your lungs a third of the way and then pause. Inhale again to fill up two thirds of the way and pause. Inhale again to fill up all the way and pause.

Exhale very slowly through your nose.

Repeat this cycle two more times.

Allow one full breath cycle without interruption.

STAGE 2: INTERRUPTED EXHALES

Inhale very slowly through your nose until your lungs are full.

Exhale a third of the breath out and then pause. Exhale two thirds of the way out and pause. Exhale the remainder of your breath and pause.

Repeat this cycle two more times.

Allow one full breath cycle without interruption.

STAGE 3: INTERRUPTED INHALES AND EXHALES

Inhale through your nose to fill up your lungs a third of the way and then pause. Inhale again to fill up two thirds of the way and pause. Inhale again to fill up all the way and pause.

Exhale a third of the breath out and pause. Exhale two thirds of the way out and pause. Exhale the remainder of your breath and pause.

Repeat this cycle two more times.

Return to a normal breath rhythm.

AFFIRMATIONS

Just like the trees that let go of their leaves in the fall, autumn teaches us to let go of what no longer serves us. This season, use these positive affirmations to connect with the essence of releasing, finding balance, and turning inward.

As you repeat these statements internally or out loud, move away from the idea that you must convince yourself of their truth. Instead, use these affirmations as a way to uncover what *is* and what *isn't* true for you. You can then make a conscious decision to focus your attention where it is needed.

1. I release all physical, emotional, and mental tension.
2. I have all the answers within me.
3. I love every cell of my body.
4. I release all worries; tomorrow is a new day.
5. I easily handle whatever comes my way.
6. I am willing to change and grow.
7. I trust my insight and intuition.
8. My inner peace is my power.
9. Every day I become more aligned with my purpose.
10. I deserve to be loved and respected.
11. My inner self always knows what to do.
12. I speak my mind with clarity and compassion.
13. I free myself from the need to be right.
14. All is well, and I am safe.
15. I am open to healing.
16. I am good enough exactly as I am.
17. I feel more at ease with every breath I take.
18. I am willing to forgive and be forgiven.
19. I feel deeply connected to my own spirit.
20. I radiate peace, love, and well-being.

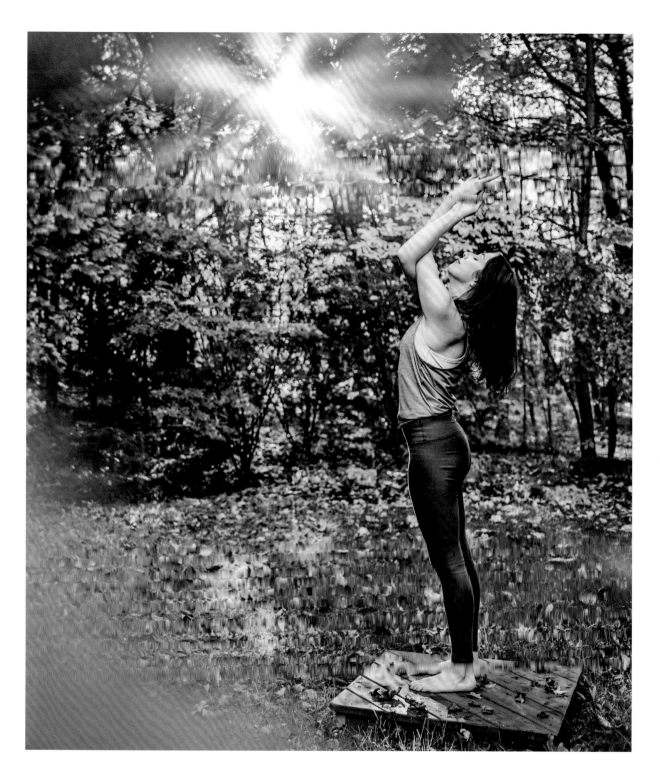

NEW MOON RITUAL

Draw a Card

Card pulls are an amazing way to connect with your subconscious mind by focusing on symbolism and intuition. You can use tarot or oracle cards for this.

To begin, choose a deck, sit in a comfortable position, and meditate for a few minutes. Clear your mind and ask for the right message to reveal itself to you. Once you're ready, open your eyes, shuffle your deck, and pick a card.

Observe your card carefully and notice what words, feelings, or thoughts come to mind when you first look at it. You may want to have a journal close by in order to note your first impressions of the card's imagery. Once you've noted your interpretation of the card, you can look up its meaning in the guide that accompanies most decks.

Ask yourself how the card you've pulled relates to the intention you'd like to set on this new moon. You can leave your card out for the month as a reminder of this intention, or place it under your pillow before going to bed.

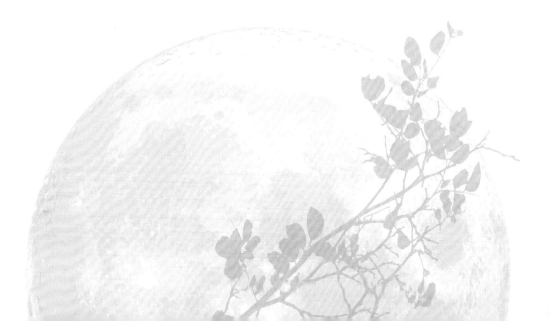

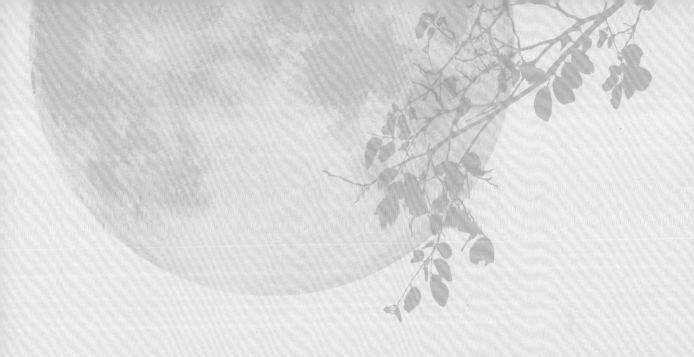

FULL MOON RITUAL

Clean House

If you're looking for an energetic cleanse, start with a physical one! The full moon represents fullness and abundance, but this abundance should be aligned with your values. True prosperity comes from finding a balance between giving and receiving.

Once a month, go through your house and see if you can find at least five things that no longer serve you. You can donate, discard, or repurpose them. Get comfortable with the idea of walking away from things, people, and situations that are not aligned with your vision and values.

You can take this one step further by doing a social media purge! Unfollow, mute, or block people and brands that don't make you feel good or that bring you down. Send them love and wish them well as you do this. Release the negative energy surrounding these relationships and make room for something new.

LISTICLE

As the wheel of the year turns, use the following recommended resources to help you elevate your morning and evening practices. You'll find a list of some of my favorite books that pair well with fall as well as tools to nurture and care for yourself.

Music

"Reflection" by Garth Stevenson
"Inner Peace" by Beautiful Chorus
"Open" by Rhye
"Only Love" by Ben Howard
"True Love" by Coldplay
"Chopping the Woods" by East Forest
"Teardrop" by Massive Attack
"River" by Ibeyi
"Full Circle" by Half Moon Run
"Always in My Head" by Coldplay
"Slow and Steady" by Of Monsters and Men
"Akaal" by Ajeet Kaur featuring Trevor Hall
"To Build a Home" by The Cinematic
    Orchestra

Books

The Dark Side of the Light Chasers by
    Debbie Ford
Light on Yoga by B. K. S. Iyengar
A New Earth by Eckhart Tolle
Seven Thousand Ways to Listen by Mark Nepo
When Things Fall Apart by Pema Chödrön
Skill in Action by Michelle Cassandra Johnson

Crystals

OBSIDIAN: This black stone is thought to protect against negativity and alleviate mental stress. It is grounding and centering.

LAPIS LAZULI: This stone is associated with enlightenment, intuition, and inner healing. It can facilitate clear communication.

DENDRITIC AGATE: Use this crystal during meditation for self-reflection and self-analysis. It can help you bring balance to the parts of yourself that need healing.

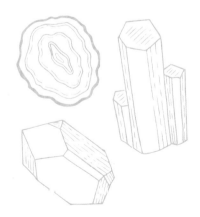

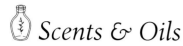 *Scents & Oils*

SANDALWOOD: A sweet and earthy scent that is deeply grounding. Often used as incense for spiritual practices.

JASMINE: A dreamy and floral aroma that is said to be an aphrodisiac.

ROSEMARY: A refreshing and stimulating scent, beneficial for alertness and mental acuity.

CHAKRA: Sacral (*Svadhisthana*)

ELEMENT: Water

MOON PHASE: Waning Moon

CARDINAL DIRECTION: West

ZODIAC: Libra, Scorpio, Sagittarius

MIXED BERRY SMOOTHIE RECIPE
SERVES 1 TO 2

1 pear, core and seeds removed

¼ cup blueberries (fresh or frozen)

½ cup pomegranate seeds (or pomegranate juice)

1 cup baby spinach

1 cup water

1 tablespoon flax seeds

½ cup ice (optional)

Combine all ingredients in a blender and add ice if desired. Blend until desired consistency is reached. You can make it creamier by replacing the water with 1 cup of any type of milk or yogurt.

YOGA SEQUENCE 1
Water Element

LEVEL: Intermediate to Advanced   **PROPS REQUIRED:** Block and strap (optional)

Fall is associated with the element of water, which is all about fluidity, sensitivity, and creativity. Water is also linked with the sacral (*Svadhisthana*) chakra located in your pelvis. This practice is all about heightening your senses and getting in touch with your emotions through deep hip openers and a fluid flow.

Working on our hips can also be a great way to release stagnant emotions. As you practice, acknowledge any feelings that may arise without judgment. Give yourself permission to go with the flow and connect with the element of water.

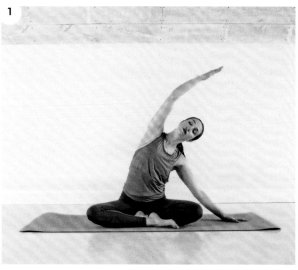

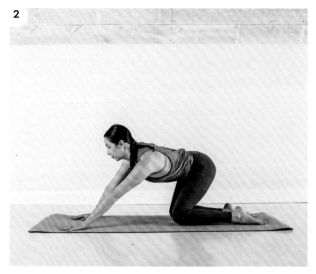

1. Seated Side Bend Pose (*Parsva Sukhasana*)

Sit comfortably in a cross-legged position with your spine tall and your shoulders down. Inhale to reach your right arm up and over into a side bend. Relax your neck and stay here for five breaths before switching to the other side.

2. Hip Circles

Come to your hands and knees and look down at the mat as you begin to trace large circles with your hips. Start by tracing them in a clockwise direction for a few rounds and then switch to counterclockwise. Press your hips all the way out to the sides and back, as if you are stirring a pot.

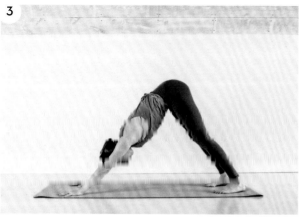

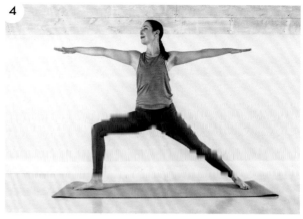

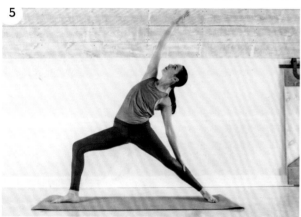

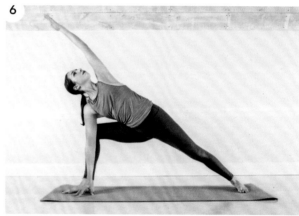

3. Downward-Facing Dog Pose

(*Adho Mukha Svanasana*)

From your hands and knees, walk your hands a few inches past your shoulders. Tuck your toes under and lift your hips up and back. Reach your chest toward your thighs and relax your neck. Hold for ten breaths.

5. Reverse Warrior Pose (*Viparita Virabhadrasana*)

Slide your left hand down your left thigh and reach your right arm up and over, coming into a side bend. Look up at your hand and keep your front thigh parallel to the mat. Hold for five breaths.

4. Warrior 2 Pose (*Virabhadrasana II*)

Step your right foot to the top of your mat and align your left foot parallel to the back of your mat. Bend your right knee generously and extend your arms out, palms facing down. Gaze over your right hand and hold for five breaths.

6. Extended Side Angle Pose

(*Utthita Parsvakonasana*)

Lower your right forearm to your right thigh, or place your hand on the mat to the inside of your right foot for an added challenge. Reach your left arm up overhead, forming a diagonal line from your left fingertips to your left foot. Hold for five breaths.

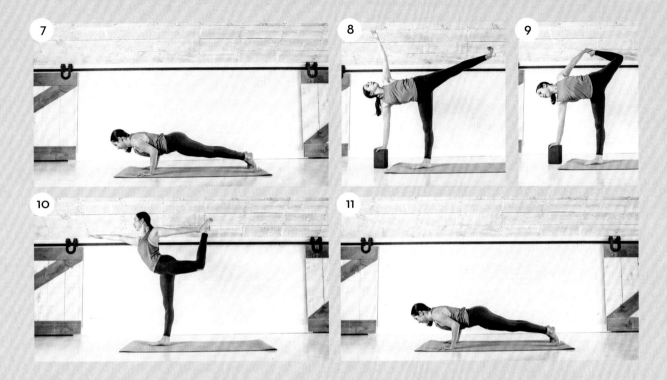

7. Vinyasa (see pages 21–22)

Place both hands down to step back into Plank pose. Flow from Plank to Four-Limbed Staff pose to Upward-Facing Dog and back to Downward-Facing Dog.

Repeat Warrior 2, Reverse Warrior, and Extended Side Angle poses on the second side. Follow with a vinyasa.

9. Sugarcane Pose (*Ardha Chandra Chapasana*)

From Half Moon pose, bend your left knee and reach back to hold your foot with your left hand. Push your foot into your palm to arch back with your spine, coming into a backbend. Hold for five breaths.

11. Vinyasa (see pages 21–22)

Release the Dancer's pose and fold forward to step back into Plank pose. Flow from Plank to Four-Limbed Staff pose to Upward-Facing Dog and back to Downward-Facing Dog.

Repeat Half Moon pose, Sugarcane pose, and Dancer's pose on the second side. Follow with a vinyasa.

8. Half Moon Pose (*Ardha Chandrasana*)

From Downward-Facing Dog pose, step your right foot forward to the top of your mat and push off your left leg to lift it up. Roll your left hip back to stack it over your right hip and reach your left arm up to the sky. You can rest your right hand on the floor or a block. Hold for five breaths.

10. Dancer's Pose (*Natarajasana*)

Maintain the hold on your left foot with your left hand and use core strength to come all the way up to standing. Balance on your right leg as you extend your right arm forward and lift your left leg up higher. Hold for five breaths.

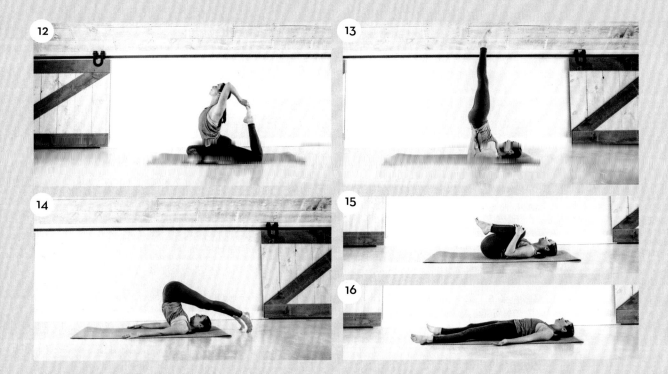

12. King Pigeon Pose (*Eka Pada Rajakapotasana*)

Place your right knee behind your right wrist and level your hips. You can place a block under your seat for more support. Bend your back knee and reach for your foot with your left hand or a strap. Pull your foot in toward you with your left hand and rotate your shoulder so your left elbow points up to the sky. Stay like this or reach your right hand back to hold on to your foot with both hands. Hold for ten breaths and step back in Downward-Facing Dog pose before switching sides.

14. Plow Pose (*Halasana*)

Lower your legs back behind you and rest your feet above your head. Straighten your legs and extend your arms flat on the floor for more support. Reach your tailbone up toward the sky. Hold for ten breaths.

16. Corpse Pose (*Savasana*)

Release the hold on your knees and stretch your arms and legs out, turning your palms toward the sky. Relax your shoulders away from your ears, close your eyes, and breathe deeply. Stay for five minutes or longer.

13. Shoulderstand Pose (*Sarvangasana*)

Lower to your back and lift your hips up high, supporting your lower back with your hands. Press your shoulders away from your neck and straighten your legs toward the sky. Create a straight line from your feet down to your hips and shoulders. Hold for ten breaths.

15. Knees-to-Chest Pose (*Apanasana*)

Slowly roll out of Plow pose to pull your knees into your chest. Press your tailbone into the ground and gently rock from side to side. Stay for ten breaths.

YOGA SEQUENCE 2
Yoga for Hamstring Flexibility

LEVEL: Intermediate to Advanced **PROPS REQUIRED:** Strap (optional)

This sequence is all about the lower part of your posterior chain—more specifically, your hamstrings. Many of us have tight hamstrings, and often, our hamstrings can also be weak and underutilized. This sequence will help you stretch and strengthen this area through some challenging reclined, seated, standing, and balancing poses.

You might notice that when you release tension from the back of your legs and learn to properly engage those muscles, you'll feel relief along your spine. The posterior chain is all connected. Remember to breathe deeply through the intensity of this flow.

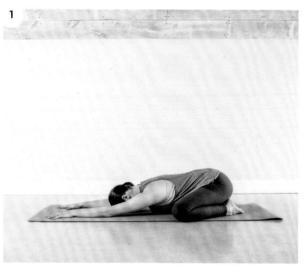

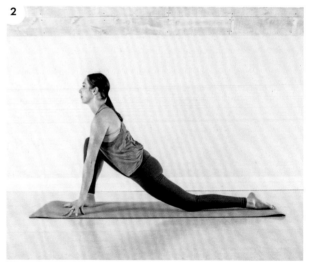

1. Extended Child's Pose
(*Utthita Balasana*)
From your hands and knees, widen your knees to the edges of your mat and bring your big toes together to touch. Press your hips back toward your heels and extend your arms forward, gently lowering your forehead to the ground. Hold for ten breaths.

2. Equestrian Pose
(*Ashwa Sanchalanasana*)
Come to your hands and knees and step your right foot forward between your palms. Align your right knee over your ankle as you melt your hips down toward the earth. Lift your chest and roll your shoulders back. Hold for five breaths.

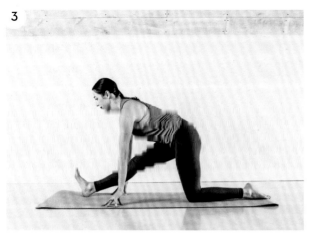

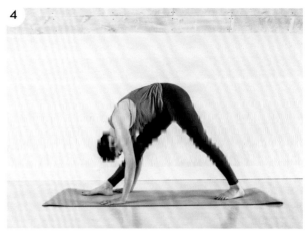

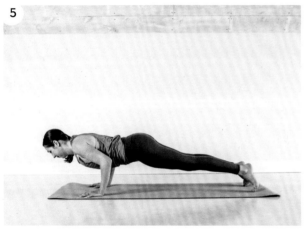

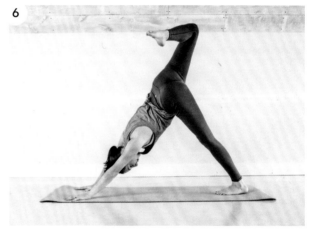

3. Half Monkey Pose

(*Ardha Hanumanasana*)

Push into your right heel to straighten your right leg and shift your hips back as you fold over your shin. Flex your front foot and press down into your heel. Hold for five breaths.

7. Vinyasa (see pages 71–77)

Bend your front knee and lower both hands down to step back into Plank pose. Flow from Plank to Four-Limbed Staff pose to Upward-Facing Dog to Downward-Facing Dog.

Repeat Equestrian, Half Monkey, and Pyramid poses on the second side. Follow with a vinyasa.

4. Pyramid Pose (*Parsvottanasana*)

Tuck the toes of your back foot under to lift your back knee off the mat. Ground your back foot at a 45-degree angle. Fold your chest down toward your right leg as you push into both feet evenly. Hold for five breaths.

6. Three-Legged Downward-Facing Dog Pose Variation (*Eka Pada Adho Mukha Svanasana*)

Lift your right leg up toward the sky and bend your knee to open your hip. Squeeze your right foot toward your seat and hold for five breaths.

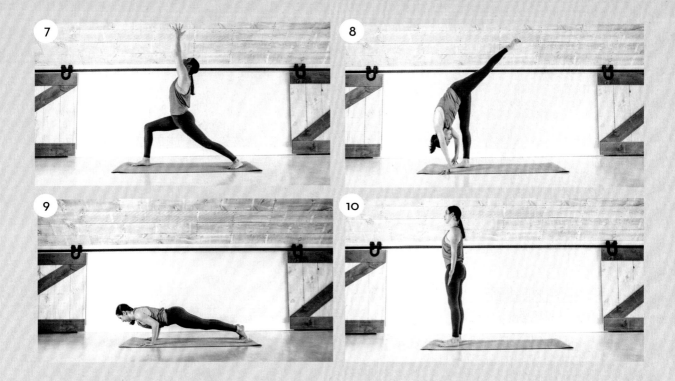

7. Warrior 1 Pose (*Virabhadrasana I*)

Step your right foot to the top of your mat and press your back heel down, placing your left foot at a 45-degree angle. Bend your front knee generously and reach your arms up overhead. Emphasize the stretch in your back leg by pushing into your heel. Hold for five breaths.

9. Vinyasa (see pages 21–22)

Bend your front knee and lower both hands down to step back into Plank pose. Flow from Plank to Four-Limbed Staff pose to Upward-Facing Dog and back to Downward-Facing Dog.

Repeat Three-Legged Downward-Facing Dog Variation, Warrior 1 pose, and Standing Splits pose on the second side. Follow with a vinyasa.

8. Standing Splits Pose (*Urdhva Prasarita Eka Padasana*)

Lower your fingertips to the floor and push off your left leg to balance on your right one. Lift your left leg up as high as it will go by engaging your glutes. Walk your hands back to bring your forehead toward your shin and hold for five breaths.

10. Mountain Pose (*Tadasana*)

Stand up tall at the top of your mat with your feet hip-width apart. Roll your shoulders back and turn your palms forward. Press into all four corners of both feet.

11. Extended Hand-to-Big-Toe Pose A (*Utthita Hasta Padangusthasana A*)

Balance on your left leg as you lift your right leg up. Hold on to your big right toe with your two peace fingers or a strap and straighten your leg in front of you as much as is comfortable. Place your left hand on your hip and straighten your spine. Hold for five breaths.

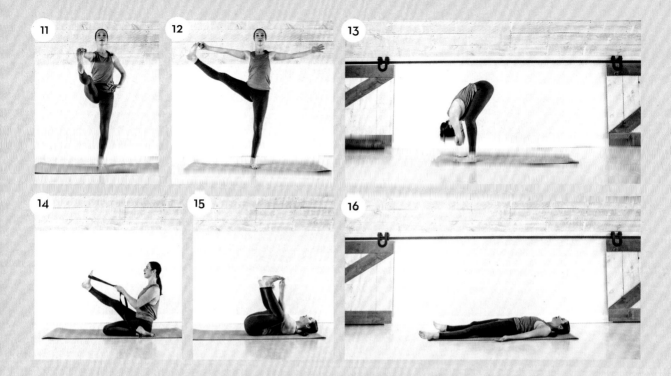

12. Extended Hand-to-Big-Toe Pose B
(*Utthita Hasta Padangusthasana B*)
Guide your right leg out to the side to externally rotate your right hip. Reach your left arm out as a counterweight. Press your right hip down as you pull on your big toe to lift your foot up. Hold for five breaths. Repeat both variations of Extended Hand-to-Big-Toe pose on the second side.

14. Heron Pose (*Krounchasana*)
Take a posture with your left leg in a kneeling position, pinning your left foot in to your right hip. Grab ahold of your right foot with your hands or a strap and extend it straight up. Roll your shoulders back and straighten your spine. Hold for ten breaths before switching sides.

16. Corpse Pose (*Savasana*)
Release the pose and extend your arms and legs out. Soften your shoulders away from your ears, face your palms upward, close your eyes, and breathe deeply. Stay for five minutes or longer.

13. Standing Forward Bend Pose Variation
(*Uttanasana*)
Place your feet slightly wider apart than your hips and fold over your legs. Bend your knees as much as is comfortable. Relax your neck and hold on to your upper arms as you sway from side to side. Hold for ten breaths.

15. Happy Baby Pose (*Ananda Balasana*)
Lower down to lie on your back. Draw your knees in toward your shoulders and press your tailbone into the floor. Stay here or progress into the full version of the pose by stacking your ankles over your knees and holding on to your big toes. Hold for ten breaths.

YOGA SEQUENCE 3
Yin Yoga for Emotional Healing

LEVEL: All Levels	**PROPS REQUIRED:** 2 blocks or a bolster

The chakras can be used as metaphors and inspiration for emotional healing and balance. This yin yoga practice invites you to dive deeper by working with the energetic body. According to yogic philosophy, the energetic body is comprised of chakras, meaning "wheels" or "discs," which allow for the flow of prana, or life force energy. Each of these energetic centers corresponds to a different theme and meaning. If you have a current issue or conflict, ask yourself how the wisdom of each chakra can help you with this dilemma. We'll do one pose per chakra working from the bottom up.

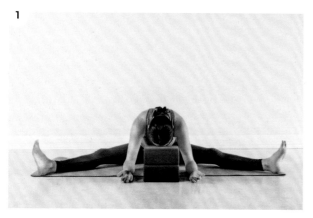

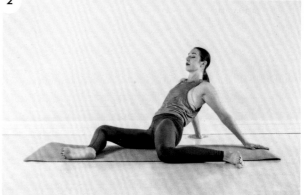

1. Straddle

Sit with your legs extended out to the sides and fold forward, walking your hands out in front of you and relaxing your arms. You can place your blocks or a bolster under your chest and forehead for more support. Hold for three to five minutes.

Focus on the first (*Muladhara*) chakra glowing bright red at the base of your spine. This relates to themes of safety, survival, family of origin, community and belonging. Visualize it healthy, healed, and whole.

2. Deer Pose

Place your right knee out in front of you at a 90-degree angle and align your left knee with your left hip, also at a 90-degree angle. Walk your hands back as far as is appropriate to stretch your inner thigh. Hold for three to five minutes before switching sides.

Focus on the second (*Svadhisthana*) chakra glowing orange in your pelvis. This relates to creativity, emotions, sexuality, and relationships. Visualize it healthy, healed, and whole.

3

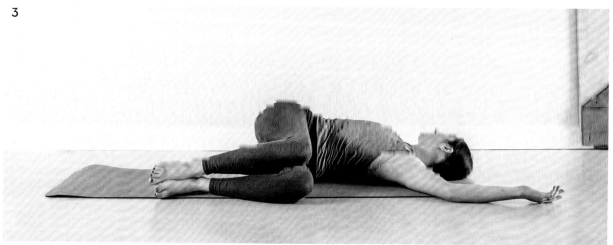

4

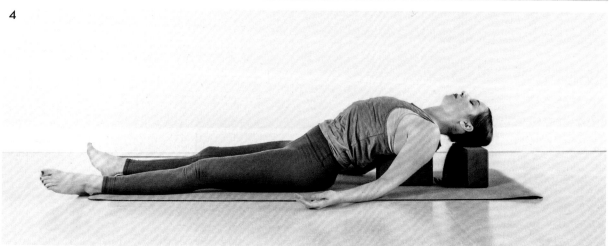

3. Lying Spinal Twist Pose

Lower onto your back and open your arms out to the sides in a cactus shape with your palms facing up. Flip your hips up and move them a few inches to the right before lowering your knees and thighs over to the left. Gaze over your right shoulder and hold for three to five minutes before repeating on the second side.

Focus on the third (*Manipura*) chakra glowing yellow above your navel. This relates to self-esteem, confidence, willpower, and determination. Visualize it healthy, healed, and whole.

4. Supported Fish Pose

Lie back on your blocks or a bolster to support your head and upper back. Bring your arms by your sides with your palms facing up and extend your legs out. Hold for three to five minutes.

Focus on the fourth (*Anahata*) chakra glowing green at your heart. This relates to compassion and love for yourself and others. Visualize it healthy, healed, and whole.

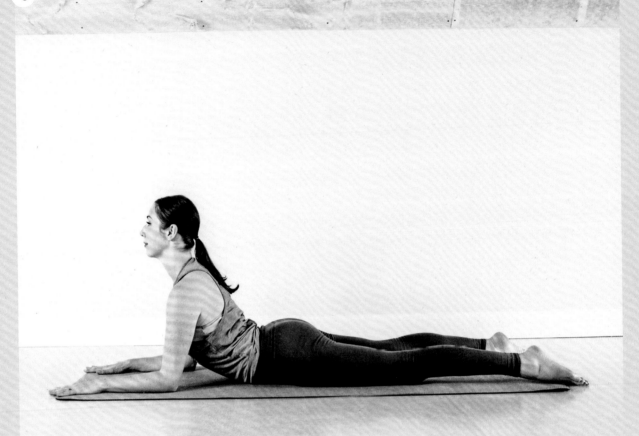

5. Sphinx Pose

Lift your chest and place your forearms flat on the mat, aligning your elbows under your shoulders. Press your shoulders back and reach your heart forward. Hold for three to five minutes.

Focus on the fifth (*Visuddha*) chakra glowing bright blue at your throat. This relates to speaking your truth, communicating clearly, and listening to others. Visualize it healthy, healed, and whole.

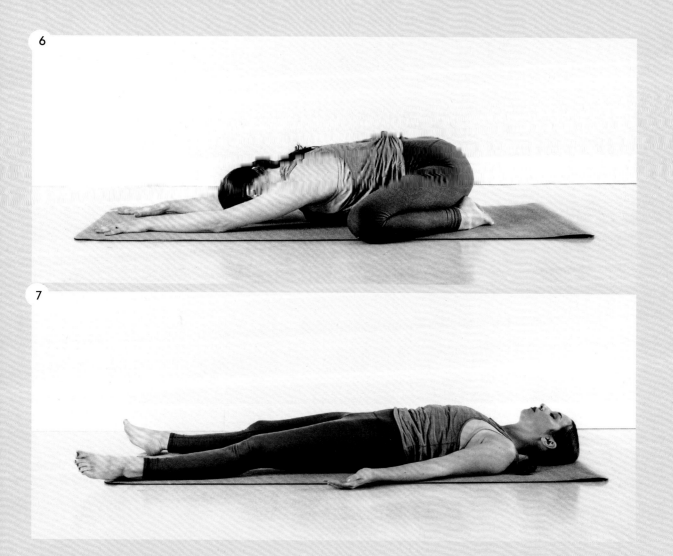

6

7

6. Child's Pose

Push back up to hands and knees and bring your big toes together [or widen both your knees with space]. Press your hips back toward your heels and walk your hands forward to melt your chest and forehead down. Hold here for three to five minutes.

Focus on the sixth (Ajna) chakra glowing indigo blue in your third eye. This relates to themes of intuition, foresight, wisdom, and guidance. Visualize it healthy, healed, and whole.

7. Corpse Pose

Lower onto your back, and extend your arms and legs out, facing your palms up toward the sky. Relax your body fully and close your eyes, holding the pose for five minutes or longer.

Finally, focus on the seventh (Sahasrara) chakra glowing violet in the crown of your head. This relates to your connection with the divine, spirituality, and oneness. Visualize it healthy, healed, and whole.

YOGA SEQUENCE 4
Yoga for Stress & Anxiety

LEVEL: Beginner   **PROPS REQUIRED:** Block and strap

Many of us carry stress in our necks, shoulders, and upper back. This beginner sequence will work on releasing tension from your upper body and soothing your nervous system with forward folds and inversions.

While you practice, emphasize slow and steady breaths that reach all the way down to your lower belly. This sequence moves at a slower pace so you can settle in each pose. At the end, you should feel relaxed and renewed.

1

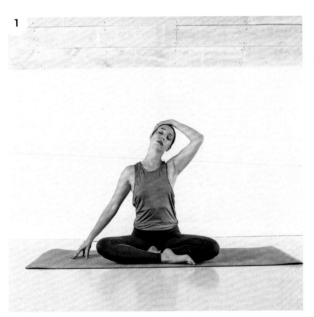

2

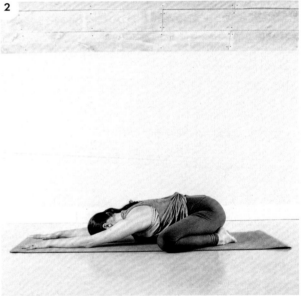

1. Seated Neck Release

Sit in Easy pose (*Sukhasana*) with your spine lifted tall. Drop your left ear to your left shoulder and slide your shoulder blades down your back. Use your left hand to pull your right ear away from your right shoulder. Take ten breaths here before switching sides.

2. Child's Pose (*Balasana*)

Come to your hands and knees and bring your big toes together to touch. Shift your hips back toward your heels and reach your arms in front of you. Rest your forehead to the mat. Hold for ten breaths.

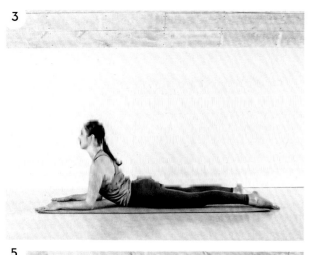

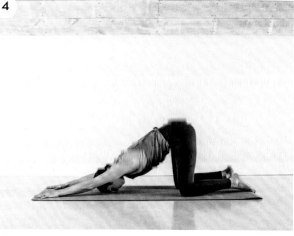

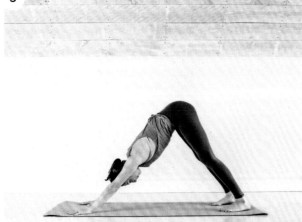

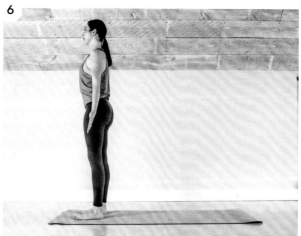

3. Sphinx Pose (*Salamba Bhujangasana*)

Lower to your belly and bring your forearms out in front of you. Lift your chest and press your pelvis into the ground. Roll your shoulders back and reach your heart forward. Hold for ten breaths.

5. Downward-Facing Dog Pose
(*Adho Mukha Svanasana*)

Tuck your toes under and lift your hips up and back. Press your hands into the ground and reach your chest toward your thighs. Relax your head and neck fully. Hold for ten breaths.

4. Puppy Pose (*Anahatasana*)

Press back up to your hands and knees and walk your hands out in front of you. Lower your forehead to the mat as you melt your heart to the ground. Keep your hips over your knees and hold for ten breaths.

6. Mountain Pose (*Tadasana*)

Walk your feet to the top of the mat and push into your heels to roll up to a standing position. Place your feet hip-width apart and your arms by your sides. Close your eyes and press down into all four corners of both feet. Hold for ten breaths.

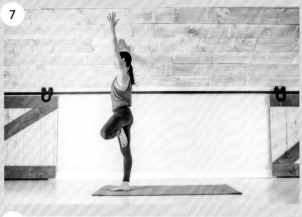

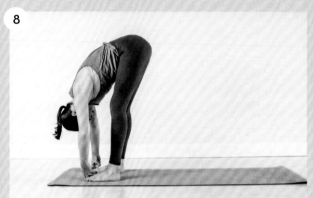

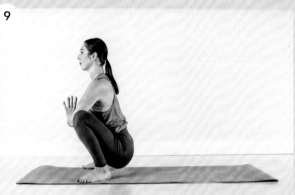

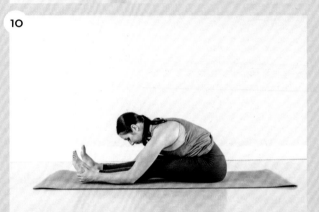

7. Tree Pose (*Vrksasana*)

Balance on your right leg and place your left foot to the inside of your right shin or right inner thigh. Engage your glutes to externally rotate your left hip. Press down into your right foot and extend your arms up overhead. Hold for ten breaths and repeat on the other side.

8. Big Toe Pose (*Padangusthasana*)

Start with your feet hip-width apart. Hinge forward at your hips to fold all the way down, bending your knees if needed. Grab your big toes with your two peace fingers and pull your elbows away from each other. Hold for ten breaths.

9. Garland Pose (*Malasana*)

Come back up to standing and point your toes out at a 45-degree angle. Sit all the way down into a squat position. Bring your hands in prayer at your heart and use your elbows to press your knees wider. Lengthen your spine and hold for ten breaths.

10. Seated Forward Bend Pose (*Paschimottanasana*)

Sit up tall with your legs extended in front of you. Inhale to reach your arms up and fold forward as you exhale, bringing your forehead toward your legs. Lengthen out of your lower back and bend your knees if needed. Hold for ten breaths.

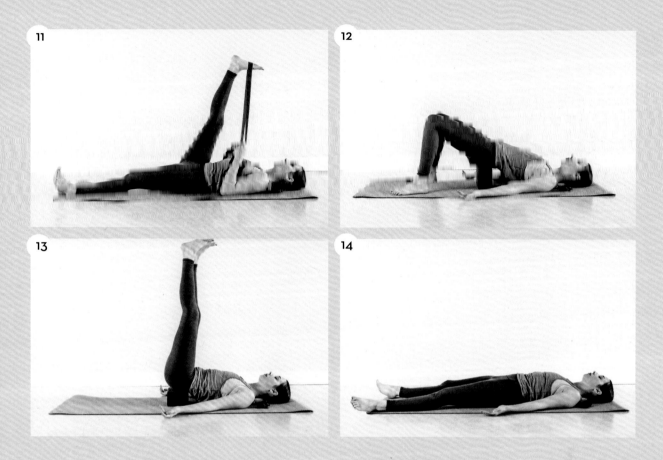

11. Reclining Hand-to-Big-Toe Pose
(*Supta Padangusthasana*)
Lie on your back with your strap in hand. Wrap the strap around the ball of your right foot as you stretch your right leg up toward the sky. Extend your left leg straight on the ground. Pull your right leg in toward you. Hold for ten breaths before switching sides.

13. Waterfall Pose (*Viparita Karani*)
Place your block on its lowest level and extend your legs up toward the sky. Keep your arms by your sides or extend them up overhead for a gentle stretch in your upper body. Let your legs dangle here for ten breaths.

12. Supported Bridge Pose
(*Setu Bandha Sarvangasana*)
Bend your knees and place your feet flat on the floor, close to your seat. Roll your shoulders away from your ears and push your feet into the ground to lift your hips up high. Grab your block and slide it under your hips at the level of your choosing. Relax your arms by your sides with your palms facing up and hold for ten breaths.

14. Corpse Pose (*Savasana*)
Release the pose and move your props out of the way. Stretch out your arms and legs and close your eyes. Turn your palms upward. Feel all tensions melt away as you stay for five minutes or longer.

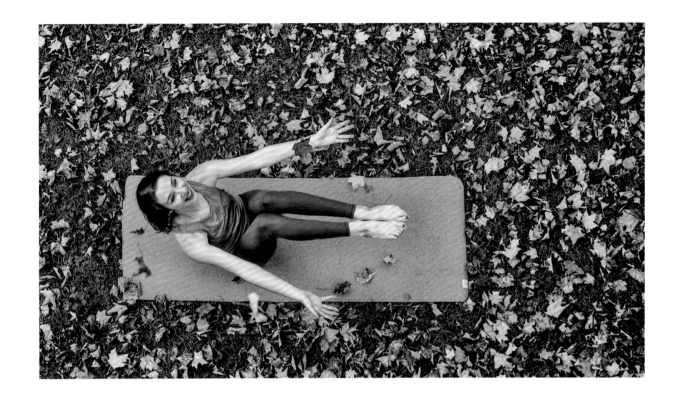

CONCLUSION

Aligning my yoga practice with the daily, lunar, and seasonal rhythms has been such a rewarding and profound journey for me. Now that we've gone through a yearlong cycle together, I hope you've noticed some positive changes in your physical, mental, emotional, and spiritual health. My wish is that this book can be an evergreen resource for you to turn to when you need an extra dose of inspiration and connection.

It has been such an honor to share this knowledge with you, and I hope you've found it both meaningful and practical. This book, with all its tools and practices, is meant to grow with you throughout the different seasons of your life and to encourage you to deepen your connection with yourself and with nature. Take what works for you and leave the rest.

From the bottom of my heart, thank you for practicing with me by reading this book, watching the video yoga classes, and listening to the audio meditations. Whichever format you chose to use, I hope it's been a worthwhile experience. Here's to the next adventure!

KReinhardt

ACKNOWLEDGMENTS

A lot of people helped bring this project to life, and I am deeply grateful for their assistance.

Thank you to my friends and family for encouraging me to push forward even when things got tough. Special recognition goes to my husband for always being my sounding board and helping me work through my ideas.

Thank you to my excellent photographer, Jessica Hodgson, for taking the most stunning shots. Shooting with you is always the best experience, and I am blown away by your talent and vision.

Big thanks to my fantastic videographer, Ivan Cooke. You're so easy to work with; you make filming for six-plus hours a day truly enjoyable!

Special thanks to my dear friend Tina Lamontagne of Yoga Attic for letting me use her gorgeous space for the indoor photos for this book. You truly know how to make a space come to life, and I am always grateful for your generosity and support.

Finally, and most important, a deep bow of gratitude to the people at Insight Editions who made this project happen.

- Katie Killebrew, Editorial Director
- Claire Yee, Editor
- Ashley Quackenbush, Associate Art Director

There simply wouldn't be a book without you, and I am eternally grateful for your expertise, guidance, creativity, and vision. Thank you for making this such a joyful and easygoing process.

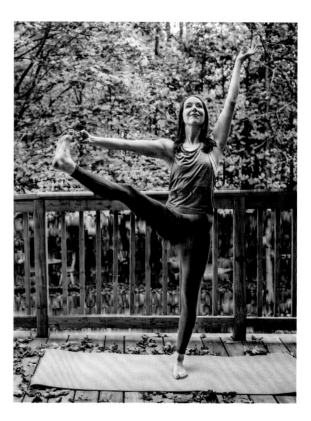

RESOURCES

Music

"Airwaves" by Ray LaMontagne

"Akaal" by Ajeet Kaur featuring Trevor Hall

"Always in My Head" by Coldplay

"As I Wake in the Morning" by Alexia Chellun

"Ascent" by Josh Brill

"Awake" by Tycho

"Beacon" by Ayla Nereo

"Blessed We Are" by Peia

"Blue Moon" by Beck

"Chimes of Peace" by Adam Lees

"Chopping the Woods" by East Forest

"Crystal" by Stevie Nicks

"Deep Peace" by Ashana

"Dreams" by Fleetwood Mac

"Every Morning" by Sugar Ray

"Faith's Hymn" by Beautiful Chorus

"Fly Like an Eagle" by Steve Miller Band

"Fly Me to the Moon" by Minnie Driver

"Flying" by Garth Stevenson

"Follow the Sun" by Xavier Rudd

"Full Circle" by Half Moon Run

"Gayatri" by Lisbeth Scott

"Goodnight Moon Child" by Beautiful Chorus

"Gravity" by John Mayer

"Green & Gold" by Lianne La Havas

"Harvest Moon" by Neil Young

"Heavy Rope (Acoustic)" by Lights

"Higher Love" by James Vincent McMorrow

"Horizon" by Garth Stevenson

"I Am Light" by India.Arie

"In My Life" by Jake Shimabukuro

"Ink" by Coldplay

"Inner Peace" by Beautiful Chorus

"Jai Ma" by Govind Das and Radha

"Lakshmi Mantra" by Jaya Lakshmi and Ananda

"Let the Drummer Kick" by Citizen Cope

"Light Me Up" by DJ Drez featuring Marti Nikko

"Lucky" by Jason Mraz and Colbie Caillat

"Lullaby" by Trevor Hall

"Mother of the Water" by Alexa Sunshine Rose

"Nectar Drop" by DJ Drez

"Om Mani Padme Hum" by Veet Vichara & Premanjali

"Only Love" by Ben Howard

"Open" by Rhye

"Opening the Heart" by Annie Jameson

"Pachamama" by Beautiful Chorus

"Peace" by Lisbeth Scott

"Please Prepare Me" by Beautiful Chorus

"Pressure" by Milk & Bone

"Purnamadah" by Shantala

"Put Your Records On" by Corinne Bailey Rae

"Reflection" by Garth Stevenson

"River" by Ibeyi

"Savasana II" by Gabriele Morgan

"Slow and Steady" by Of Monsters and Men

"Slowly" by Max Sedgley

"Small Memory" by Jon Hopkins

"Sound of Invisible Waters" by Deuter

"Surya Namaskar (Sun Salutation)" by Michael Mandrell and Benjy Wertheimer

"Teardrop" by Massive Attack

"The Mountain" by Trevor Hall

"The Sound of Silence" by Pat Metheny

"The Southern Sea" by Garth Stevenson

"Thula Nana 'Tula" by Thula Nana

"To Build a Home" by The Cinematic Orchestra

"True Love" by Coldplay

"Veiled Grey" by Christian Löffler

"When I Get My Hands on You" by The New Basement Tapes

"Window" by The Album Leaf

"Winter Birds" by Ray LaMontagne

"Wish You Were Here" by Pink Floyd

Books

A New Earth by Eckhart Tolle

A Return to Love by Marianne Williamson

Awakening Shakti by Sally Kempton

Being Mortal by Atul Gawande

Embrace Yoga's Roots by Susanna Barkataki

Light on Yoga by B. K. S. Iyengar

Living Your Yoga by Judith Hanson Lasater

Lunar Abundance by Ezzie Spencer

Man's Search for Meaning by Viktor Frankl

Meditations from the Mat by Rolf Gates

Moon Time by Lucy H. Pearce

Moonology by Yasmin Boland

Radical Acceptance by Tara Brach

Seven Thousand Ways to Listen by Mark Nepo

Siddhartha by Hermann Hesse

Skill in Action by Michelle Cassandra Johnson

Tantra Illuminated by Christopher Wallis

The Bhagavad Gita by the sage Vyasa

The Dark Side of the Light Chasers by Debbie Ford

The Power Map by Danielle LaPorte

The Heart of Yoga by T. K. V. Desikachar

The Mastery of Love by Don Miguel Ruiz

The Untethered Soul by Michael A. Singer

The Yoga of the Nine Emotions by Peter Marchand

The Yoga Sutras of Patanjali by Sri Swami Satchidananda

When Things Fall Apart by Pema Chödrön

Women Who Run with the Wolves by Clarissa Pinkola Estés

Year of Yes by Shonda Rhimes

Yoga Poems by Leza Lowitz

You Can Heal Your Life by Louise Hay

Crystals

AMETHYST: This crystal will help you tap into your imagination and give you a boost of inspiration. It has calming properties and can help improve the quality of your sleep and the vividness of your dreams.

AQUAMARINE: Balance the heat of summer with this cool and calm stone that represents cloudy waters. Think of it as your "go with the flow" ally.

AVENTURINE: Think of this as your good-luck charm! As you move forward with your dreams and goals, aventurine supports you in forward positive action. Use this stone when taking risks.

BLACK TOURMALINE: This crystal represents the darkness of the new moon. Use this stone to uncover hidden parts of yourself. It can be used for deep healing and grounding.

CARNELIAN: This stone is said to boost creativity and vitality. It offers healing energy and gives us the courage to try something new.

CITRINE: This is the crystal of abundance! Citrine is also associated with confidence and the solar plexus (*Manipura*) chakra. Its orange color is reminiscent of the sun.

CLEAR QUARTZ: When it comes to setting intentions, clear quartz is the way to go! This stone amplifies energy and clarifies your thoughts. It is sometimes referred to as the master healer.

DENDRITIC AGATE: Use this crystal during meditation for self-reflection and self-analysis. It can help you bring balance to the parts of yourself that need healing.

LABRADORITE: Use this stone to tap into your creativity and deepest desires. When setting intentions, this crystal can help you see the bigger picture.

LAPIS LAZULI: This stone is associated with enlightenment, intuition, and inner healing. It can facilitate clear communication.

MOONSTONE: This crystal can help you tap into your highest vision and intuition. It is also thought to bring about good dreams.

OBSIDIAN: This black stone is thought to protect against negativity and alleviate mental stress. It is grounding and centering.

RED JASPER: Connected to the root (*Muladhara*) chakra, this stone helps you feel grounded and secure so that you can tap into your own inner power.

ROSE QUARTZ: This stone is closely related to the heart (*Anahata*) chakra. It helps us connect to love and compassion and helps us have an open heart. The soft pink color is also reminiscent of cherry blossoms and other spring flowers.

SELENITE: Named after the ancient Greek goddess of the moon, Selene, selenite is the perfect full moon ally. It is an energetic cleanser connected to higher consciousness.

SUNSTONE: Associated with vitality and joy, this crystal is thought to bring goodwill and optimism.

Scents & Oils

CEDARWOOD: If you're feeling frazzled or distracted, cedarwood can help ground you and calm your nerves.

CINNAMON. This is an invigorating scent that captures the fiery spirit of the summer season.

CITRONELLA: This refreshing and uplifting scent has the added benefit of being an insect repellent.

CLOVE: Use this scent for warmth and relaxation. Traditionally, this is thought to be a health booster, specifically for the respiratory and digestive systems.

EUCALYPTUS: Use this scent for a boost of energy and invigoration. It supports easy breathing and can lift your mood during the darkest winter days.

FRANKINCENSE: Use this oil as an accompaniment during meditation to facilitate spiritual connection. It is both uplifting and grounding.

GRAPEFRUIT. Refresh your senses and gain mental clarity with this citrus scent.

JASMINE: A dreamy and floral aroma that is said to be an aphrodisiac.

LAVENDER: Use this soothing scent when you need to calm down and relax.

NEROLI: Use this floral scent to evoke peaceful and soothing energy.

PEPPERMINT: Get a boost of energy and clear away brain fog with the invigorating peppermint scent.

ROSEMARY: A refreshing and stimulating scent beneficial for alertness and mental acuity.

SAGE: Sage has long been regarded as an energetically cleansing plant by various cultures around the world, from the ancient Romans to the Celts and Indigenous populations across North America. Use it for new beginnings and to shift your mood.

SANDALWOOD: A sweet and earthy scent that is deeply grounding. Often used as incense for spiritual practices.

VANILLA: Embrace the vibrancy and sensuality of the full moon with this natural aphrodisiac. Vanilla can also be a mood booster.

YLANG YLANG: Use this scent to connect with your divine feminine energy. It also relates to romance and joy.

INDEX

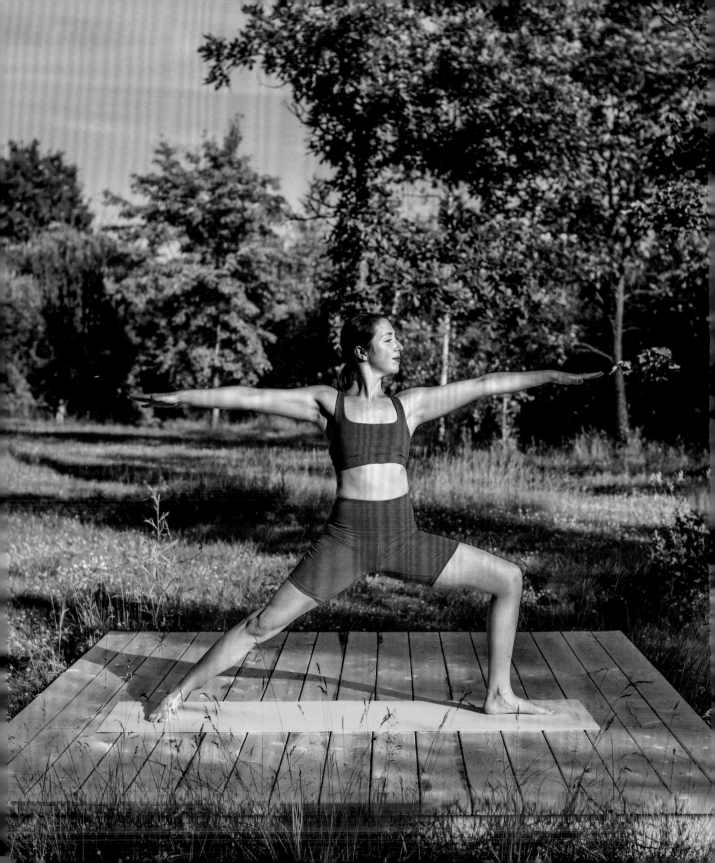

ABOUT THE AUTHOR

Kassandra Reinhardt, author of *Yin Yoga: Stretch the Mindful Way*, is an Ottawa-based yoga instructor on a mission to help others feel great with yoga! She first began taking classes in 2008 as a way to become more flexible and manage stress and anxiety. She fell in love with the richness of her yoga practice and wanted to share it with others. A yoga teacher since 2012, she has completed two-hundred–and three-hundred–hour yoga teacher trainings and has certifications in yin yoga and yoga therapy. Her teaching style is creative and precise. She believes that doing just a little bit of yoga every day can change your life.

Reinhardt has been featured in *Shape Magazine*, *Elite Daily*, and *ELLE Australia* and on MTV UK and CBC News. She runs international yoga retreats and offers online continuing education programs for yoga instructors who want to deepen their knowledge.

She started her Yoga with Kassandra YouTube channel in 2014, which has become one of the largest in the wellness space, with over 1.8 million subscribers and 140 million views. It has served as the gateway for millions of people around the globe to discover the life-changing benefits of vinyasa and yin yoga. She is best known for her yin yoga classes and her ten-minute morning yoga sequences. Practice with her today and browse through her growing library of free online classes at www.yogawithkassandra.com.

MANDALA

an imprint of Insight Editions
P.O. Box 3088
San Rafael, CA 94912
www.MandalaEarth.com

ISBN: 978-1-68188-845-3
Printed in China
First printed in 2022

CEO Raoul Goff

ASSOCIATE PUBLISHER Phillip Jones

EDITORIAL DIRECTOR Katie Killebrew

VP CREATIVE Chrissy Kwasnik

VP MANUFACTURING Alix Nicholaeff

ASSOCIATE ART DIRECTOR Ashley Quackenbush

EDITOR Claire Yee

PRODUCTION MANAGER Greg Steffen

PRODUCTION ASSOCIATE Deena Hashem

SR PRODUCTION MANAGER, SUBSIDIARY RIGHTS Lina s Palma

Weldon Owen would also like to thank Rachel Anderson,
Michael Clark, and Kevin Broccoli.

ROOTS of PEACE · REPLANTED PAPER

Mandala Publishing, in association with Roots of Peace, will plant two trees for each tree used in the manufacturing of this book. Roots of Peace is an internationally renowned humanitarian organization dedicated to eradicating land mines worldwide and converting war-torn lands into productive farms and wildlife habitats. Roots of Peace will plant two million fruit and nut trees in Afghanistan and provide farmers there with the skills and support necessary for sustainable land use.